THIRD
EDITION

Differentiated Instructional Strategies

One Size Doesn't Fit All

OTHER CORWIN BOOKS BY GAYLE H. GREGORY & CAROLYN CHAPMAN

Differentiated Literacy Strategies for English Language Learners, Grades K–6
by Gayle H. Gregory and Amy Burkman, 2012

Differentiated Literacy Strategies for English Language Learners, Grades 7–12
by Gayle H. Gregory and Amy Burkman, 2012

The Best of Corwin: Differentiated Instruction
by Gayle H. Gregory, 2010

Differentiated Instructional Strategies for the Block Schedule
by Gayle H. Gregory and Lynne E. Herndon, 2010

Student Teams That Get Results: Teaching Tools for the Differentiated Classroom
by Gayle H. Gregory and Lin Kuzmich, 2010

Differentiated Instructional Strategies in Practice: Training, Implementation, and Supervision
by Gayle H. Gregory, 2009

Activities for The Differentiated Classroom Series: Kindergarten Through Grade 5
by Gayle H. Gregory and Carolyn Chapman, 2008

Activities for the Differentiated Classroom: Language Arts, Grades 6–8
by Gayle H. Gregory and Carolyn Chapman, 2008

Differentiated Instructional Strategies in Practice:
Training, Implementation, and Supervision, 2e
by Gayle H. Gregory, 2008

Differentiated Instructional Strategies for Science, Grades K–8
by Gayle H. Gregory and Elizabeth Hammerman, 2008

Activities for the Differentiated Classroom: Math, Grades 6–8
by Gayle H. Gregory and Carolyn Chapman, 2008

Activities for the Differentiated Classroom: Science, Grades 6–8
by Gayle H. Gregory and Carolyn Chapman, 2008

Teacher Teams That Get Results:
61 Group Process Skills and Strategies
by Gayle H. Gregory and Lin Kuzmich, 2007

Designing Brain Compatible Learning (Third Edition)
by Gayle H. Gregory and Terence Parry, 2006

Differentiating Instruction With Style:
Aligning Teacher and Learner Intelligences for Maximum Achievement
by Gayle H. Gregory, 2005

Differentiated Assessment Strategies:
One Tool Doesn't Fit All
by Carolyn Chapman and Rita King, 2004

Differentiated Literacy Strategies for Student Growth and Achievement in Grades 7–12
by Gayle H. Gregory and Lin Kuzmich, 2005

Differentiated Literacy Strategies for Student Growth and Achievement in Grades K–6
by Gayle H. Gregory and Lin Kuzmich, 2004

Data Driven Differentiation in the Standards-Based Classroom
by Gayle H. Gregory and Lin Kuzmich, 2004

Differentiated Instructional Strategies for Reading in the Content Areas
by Carolyn Chapman and Rita King, 2003

Differentiated Instructional Strategies for Writing in the Content Areas
by Carolyn Chapman and Rita King, 2003

Gayle H. Gregory | Carolyn Chapman

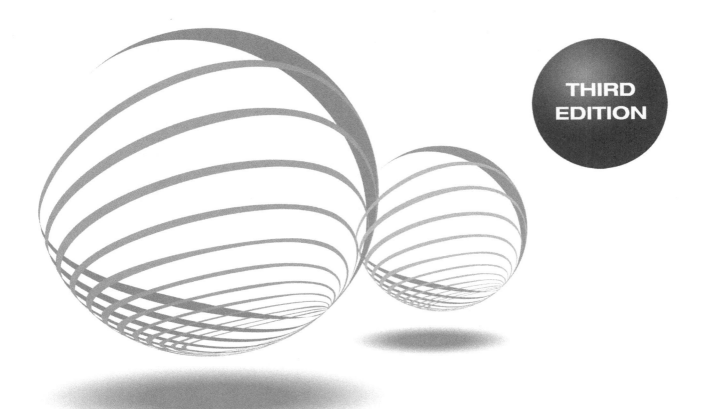

THIRD EDITION

Differentiated Instructional Strategies

One Size Doesn't Fit All

CORWIN
A SAGE Company

CORWIN
A SAGE Company

FOR INFORMATION:

Corwin
A SAGE Company
2455 Teller Road
Thousand Oaks, California 91320
(800) 233-9936
www.corwin.com

SAGE Publications Ltd.
1 Oliver's Yard
55 City Road
London EC1Y 1SP
United Kingdom

SAGE Publications India Pvt. Ltd.
B 1/I 1 Mohan Cooperative Industrial Area
Mathura Road, New Delhi 110 044
India

SAGE Publications Asia-Pacific Pte. Ltd.
3 Church Street
#10-04 Samsung Hub
Singapore 049483

Acquisitions Editor: Jessica Allan
Editorial Assistant: Lisa Whitney
Production Editor: Libby Larson
Copy Editor: Sarah J. Duffy
Typesetter: C&M Digitals (P) Ltd.
Proofreader: Theresa Kay
Indexer: Judy Hunt
Cover Designer: Rose Storey
Graphic Designer: Cristina Kubota

Printed in the United States of America.

A catalog record of this book is available from the Library of Congress.

ISBN 978-1-4522-6098-3

This book is printed on acid-free paper.

12 13 14 15 16 10 9 8 7 6 5 4 3 2 1

Content Overview

material taught and are assigned a challenging, engaging experience to learn more information. Students master information and develop skills at different times, so individual and group assignments are planned to be fluid and flexible. This chapter shares the acronym TAPS for helping with flexible grouping, representing **T**otal or whole-group instruction, **A**lone or independent work, **P**artner tasks, and **S**mall-group assignments.

One Size Doesn't Fit All!

Detailed Contents

Preface

We wrote *Differentiated Instructional Strategies: One Size Doesn't Fit All* as a useful practical, organized, and comprehensive resource to meet the diverse needs of learners. We are seasoned teachers with many years of experience working in the classroom and with adult learners all around the world. The first edition, published in 2001, connected current practice to the evolution of the teaching and learning profession. The second edition followed in 2007. With all of the recent and emerging educational issues and research, we felt a compelling need to update this well-used and well-received book. Initially, we wrote the book to bring together the various facets and concepts that were espoused as differentiation, and also to show what to do in the classroom by incorporating research and best practices from neuroscience, assessment, and education in instruction. We hoped that it would be a one-stop resource for both beginning and experienced educators.

Differentiated Instructional Strategies offers the advantage of not only simplicity, but also practicality. We put the pieces of the differentiation puzzle together, rather than just presenting a group of strategies and unpacking the "mystery" of differentiation. We highlight research relating to many concepts and provide a comprehensive framework that outlines all of the elements in a differentiated classroom, including creating climate, knowing the learner, assessments, instructional best practices, and curriculum models. We explain the strategies and concepts with examples in a teacher-friendly way that can be used from prekindergarten through Grade 12.

We have added strategies to reach more learners through engagement and choice. The framework we provide can be an overview from which expertise can be celebrated and new challenges targeted for continuous teacher improvement and growth in order to reach more learners. We also provide a lesson or unit planning template that enables teachers to create plans based on the Common Core State Standards (CCSS) while differentiating based on students' readiness, interests, and preferences.

In this third edition we have added new information, issues, and challenges to make it a richer resource for teachers, teacher leaders, professional learning communities, and administrators.

Clarity in terms of 21st century skills and the emergence in the United States of the CCSS help us as educators focus on the curriculum with the end in mind. We are realizing that we are not educating our students for a test but rather for life. We have infused our instruction with acceleration, critical thinking, equity, and support (ACES) to provide the best opportunities for students, and we have embedded the skills of collaboration, problem solving, and creative and critical thinking.

For 30 years we have watched as neuroscience has influenced educators to create safe and brain-friendly classrooms, and neuroscience is continuing to have an impact on teachers, students, and the classroom. Although brain research was noted in the two previous editions, we have tried to be more explicit about neuroscience and its connections to differentiation and student learning. We have incorporated information from works such as Dweck's (2006) *Mindsets* into this edition to help teachers create a safe, brain-friendly, differentiated classroom where they work with students to develop a *growth mindset*.

As teachers work collaboratively to focus on targeting standards, they are also aware of the unique differences in their students and the need to adjust, accommodate, and differentiate. Although there is no quantitative research to support the effectiveness of teaching to learning styles and multiple intelligences, we know people learn and prefer to learn in different ways on different days. With this in mind, we suggest that learning profiles be compiled, especially for hard-to-serve students, and that they take into account many facets of students' interests and needs, including gender and cultural issues.

Our hope is that this book serves you as a rich resource for assisting teachers and students to be the best they can be.

Acknowledgments

Corwin gratefully acknowledges the contributions of the following reviewers:

Kathleen Chamberlain
Assistant Professor of Education
Lycoming College
Williamsport, PA

Sarah Rees Edwards
Adjunct Professor
University of Arizona
Tucson, AZ

Steve Hutton
Educational Consultant, Highly Skilled Educator Program
Kentucky Department of Education
Villa Hills, KY

Rita S. King
Educational Consultant and Adjunct Professor, Department of Educational Leadership
Middle Tennessee State University
Murfreesboro, TN

Lin Kuzmich
Educational Consultant
KCS, Inc.
Loveland, CO

Mildred Murray-Ward
Chair, Department of Advanced Studies
California Lutheran University
Thousand Oaks, CA

Maria Elena Reyes
Assistant Professor, School of Education
University of Alaska
Fairbanks, AK

About the Authors

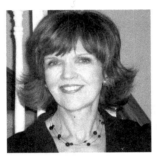

Gayle H. Gregory has been a teacher in elementary, middle, and secondary schools. For many years, she taught in schools with extended periods of instructional time (block schedules). She has had extensive districtwide experience as a curriculum consultant and staff development coordinator. She was course director at York University for the Faculty of Education, teaching in the teacher education program. She now consults internationally (Europe, Asia, North and South America, Australia) with teachers, administrators, and staff developers in the areas of brain-compatible learning, block scheduling, emotional intelligence, instructional and assessment practices, cooperative group learning, presentation skills, renewal of secondary schools, enhancing teacher quality, coaching and mentoring, and managing change. She is the author and coauthor of many books including *Teacher Teams That Get Results, Differentiated Instructional Strategies in Practice, Differentiating Instruction With Style, Data-Driven Differentiation in the Standards-Based Classroom, Differentiated Literacy Strategies for Student Growth and Achievement in Grades K–6, Differentiated Literacy Strategies for Student Growth and Achievement in Grades 7–12, Differentiated Literacy Strategies for English Language Learners, Grades K–6, Differentiated Literacy Strategies for English Language Learners, Grades 7–12, Differentiated Instructional Strategies for the Block Schedule, Teacher Teams That Get Results: 61 Group Process Skills and Strategies, Student Teams That Get Results: 61 Group Process Skills and Strategies, What Principals Should Know About Differentiation,* and *Think Big, Start Small: How to Differentiate Instruction in a Brain-Friendly Classroom.* She has been featured in *Video Journal of Education*'s editions on differentiated instruction and *Teacher Teams That Get Results.* She is committed to lifelong learning and professional growth for herself and others. She may be contacted by calling (716) 698-8716 or by e-mail at gregorygayle@ netscape.net. Her website is www.gaylehgregory.com.

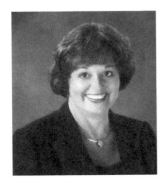

Carolyn Chapman continues her life's goal as an international professional developer, author, and teacher. She supports educators in their process of change for today's students. She has taught in a variety of settings, from kindergarten to college classrooms. Her interactive, hands-on, professional development opportunities focus on challenging the mind to ensure success for learners of all ages. In her books and her professional development opportunities, participants are engaged in exciting active learning that puts theory into practice. She walks her walk and talks her talk to make a difference in the journey of learning in today's classrooms. Carolyn feels the urgency to be a messenger and a cheerleader for educators as she watches, listens and studies effective teachers at work in classrooms. Educators are the experts because they work daily to make a difference for students. Teachers have to find that key to reach that individual learner. It is an important part of her life to provide tools, strategies, techniques, and ideas that can make a difference for students to learn.

She has authored and coauthored a number of books and publications. In addition to her writing experience, Corwin Press and School Improvement Network have featured her in several multimedia resources on differentiated instruction. Her book publications include *Differentiated Instructional Strategies: One Size Doesn't Fit All, Differentiated Assessment Strategies: One Tool Doesn't Fit All, Test Success in the Brain- Compatible Classroom, Differentiated Instructional Strategies for Reading in the Content Areas, Differentiated Instructional Strategies for Writing in the Content Areas, If the Shoe Fits: How to Develop Multiple Intelligences in the Classroom, Multiple Assessments for Multiple Intelligences, and Multiple Intelligences Through Centers and Projects.* Her company, Creative Learning Connection, Inc. has produced a CD, Carolyn Chapman's Making the Shoe Fit, and published training manuals based on each of her books. Each of these publications demonstrates her desire and determination to make an effective impact for educators and students.

At the present time, she is living in St. Helena Island, South Carolina. She continues to write while teaching courses, conducting professional development trainings, keynoting and presenting at conferences, and working on-site in long-term relationships with schools, states, and districts to provide professional development opportunities.

Carolyn may be contacted by calling (843) 838-0235 or (706) 830-0621. Her current email address is cjchapman52@gmail.com

1

One Size Doesn't Fit All

CLASSROOMS ARE FULL OF DIVERSE LEARNERS IN THIS SECOND DECADE of the 21st century, both culturally and linguistically (Goodwin, Lefkowits, Woempner, & Hubbell, 2011). Each student is unique. They differ in countless ways, including physical characteristics, personalities, backgrounds, cognitive abilities, experiences, learning preferences, and social development. Teaching experience and recent research tell us each brain is distinctively wired and impacted by previous experiences. With this knowledge, effective teachers know that learners cannot be placed through the same education hoops. Experience and research continue to provide insights about the human brain. Each student is different, they have had exclusive opportunities, and their brains are wired uniquely. So it's only reasonable that everyone learns differently and has different likes, interests, preferences, and needs.

Students bring their interests, personal experiences, and attitudes to each learning moment of every day in a classroom. How does a teacher reach the diverse needs in a classroom today? See each class member as a valuable star! All learners bring differing prior knowledge and skills. To develop deep understanding, they need not only factual but conceptual knowledge. Customized teaching and learning benefits all students with effective lessons that meet the individual needs of each learner. To emphasize this point, consider the purchase of school uniforms. Each one is sized and adjusted for the student's fit and comfort. With this in mind, we can routinely remind ourselves to differentiate instruction because "one size doesn't fit all"!

Yet for years we have planned "The Lesson" and taught it to all, knowing that we were boring some and losing others because they were not ready for that learning. Still, we expect students to adjust to the learning when the learning should really be adjusted to the learners. Adjustments should be based on sound knowledge of the learners. This includes what they know already, can do, like, are like, need, and prefer.

Effective teachers must be familiar with both their students and the Common Core State Standards (CCSS) or standards in their district or county and the students

Figure 1.1   As With Clothing, So With Lessons: One Size Does Not Fit All

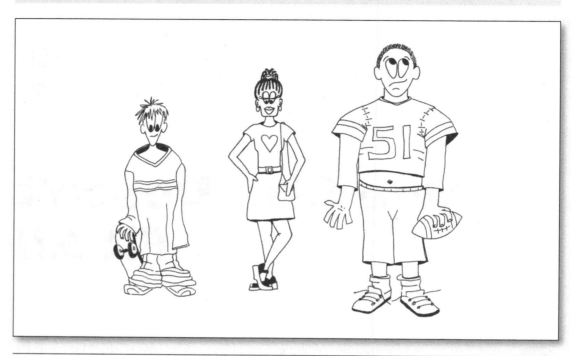

they teach. The Common Core State Standards were developed to give a national consistency rather than differing standards state to state. They were also designed to be clearer, go deeper, and prepare students to become critical and creative thinkers, college or career ready in a global market. The standards and the needs of students should determine instructional decisions. Programs, materials, and resources should not determine the curriculum and instruction. Specific materials and resources are selected to teach to the needs of the particular group of students and the standards being addressed.

Our quest in schools and classrooms everywhere as well as in the CCSS is to foster success for students in their lives by becoming self-directed, productive problem solvers and thinkers. For years, we have been studying and implementing research and evidence-based instructional strategies and assessment tools that make a difference in student achievement. *Differentiation* is a philosophy or mindset that enables educators to plan strategically in order to reach the needs of the diverse learners in classrooms today so that they can achieve targeted standards. Differentiation is not a set of tools, but a belief system or mindset that educators embrace to meet the unique needs of every learner.

The mindset of teachers who are differentiating in their classrooms embraces the following ideas:

- All students have areas of strength.
- All students have areas that need to be strengthened.
- Each student's brain is as unique as a fingerprint.

- It is never too late to learn.
- When beginning a new topic, students bring their prior knowledge base and experience to the learning.
- Emotions, feelings, and attitudes affect learning.
- All students can learn.
- Students learn in different ways at different times.

By using a variety of differentiated instructional strategies and activities, educators are implementing this philosophy daily in classrooms across the grade levels and content areas. Each time a teacher meets the individual needs of a student, he or she is differentiating instruction.

Differentiating instruction is not new, but it requires a more conscious effort on the teacher's part to analyze available data and make decisions about what is working and what needs to be adjusted. Keep what works. Discard practices that do not work. Change what needs changing. Educators are already doing a great job! More conscious consideration and a greater repertoire of strategies will help them do an even better job.

A 2007 report issued by the National Institute of Child Health and Human Development says that "aspects of development—neural, cognitive, social, psychological, physical and ethical—*have far-reaching effects on children's ability to learn. . . .* [Teachers] need access to scientifically-based knowledge concerning student development and learning."

THE DIFFERENTIATED CLASSROOM

A *differentiated classroom* is one in which the teacher responds to the unique needs of students. Carol Ann Tomlinson (1999) names content, process, and products as components that are differentiated in a classroom. The content is what is taught. The way a learner interprets, adapts, and finds ownership is the process. The product shows the learner's personal interpretation and what he or she knows. Each of these components is constantly assessed to create quality plans to meet the individual needs of students. Differentiated instruction offers a variety of options for successfully reaching the targeted standards in the CCSS. It meets learners where they are and offers challenging, appropriate options for them in order to achieve success.

Teachers can strategically and effectively differentiate the following:

- content
- assessment tools
- performance tasks
- instructional strategies

Differentiating Content

The first step is deciding which Common Core State Standards are to be targeted. Then essential questions are composed and the knowledge, skills, and understandings are highlighted. Depending on the readiness and interests of the students, the content may be differentiated. Teachers also have the added tools available in the CCSS that allow them to look at the learning progressions related to the standards so that they know what students have been exposed to and what skills they will need at the next grade level. The information to teach and the resources to best teach it are selected strategically. This is implemented by

- using different genres,
- leveling materials,
- using a variety of instructional materials,
- providing choice, and
- using selective abandonment.

Quality differentiated content is relevant to the study, interesting and intriguing to learners, has a defined purpose, and has established learning goals that target the identified Common Core State Standards. The planned assignments are not boring or frustrating, but challenging and timely for learners and will clearly show the student's competency related to the targeted standards. A wide variety of materials and resources need to be accessible for students to explore, discover, and expand their knowledge of the content. The key is selecting the most effective cognitive opportunities that are relevant, engaging, and challenging to ensure learning for each student.

Differentiating Formative Assessment Tools

Many teachers are already effectively differentiating assessment during and after the learning. However, it is equally important to assess knowledge and interests prior to the learning. Understanding what students know about the upcoming topic is essential to planning quality learning experiences. Dispense a blending of formal and informal tools for ongoing formative assessment throughout the learning experience. It is important to interpret the gathered data and use the learned information to plan strategically to meet learners' individual needs. This important learned information determines what to teach and whether interventions or more challenging learning opportunities are needed for individual learners.

Types of formative assessment include a collection of formal and informal tools that are strategically chosen to assess before, during, and after the learning. Teachers are constantly adding new ways to assess levels of understanding and needs. Use the gathered data to plan differentiated instruction to meet the diverse needs of learners.

Differentiating Performance Tasks

Students demonstrate their knowledge in many different ways. Teachers should provide various authentic opportunities and choices for learners to show what they know. For example, students can choose how to demonstrate their knowledge by creating a prop, giving an oral report, or engaging in a center experience.

Differentiating Instructional Strategies

When teachers vary instructional strategies and activities, more students learn content and information, and they develop the necessary skills. By targeting diverse intelligences and learning preferences, teachers can label learning activities and assignments in ways that help students choose when to work with their areas of strength and when to work with areas that still need strengthening. Providing options or choices enables students to learn the material their way or show what they have learned. Using research-based best practices (Dean, Hubbell, Pitler, & Stone, 2012) will help ensure that more students develop the concepts and skills targeted. Rehearsal in a variety of ways helps learning become part of long-term memory.

As with clothing, one size doesn't fit all, so in classrooms one way is not the only way.

WHY DIFFERENTIATE?

We have been faced with more change than ever before in education. Several decades ago, teachers came into the profession with a desire to work with children, a knowledge base, and good intentions. Today, teachers face a challenging landscape that is in constant flux. Many factors influence the constantly changing classroom:

- CCSS-based classrooms: targeted expectations set by states, provinces, and/or nations
- High expectations for all students: no longer can we leave children behind and just "spray and pray" for success
- Multicultural diversity: continuous influx of immigrant children with little or no communication skills or competencies in English
- Student diversity: unique learning preferences and different strengths of multiple intelligences
- New cognitive research on human learning: knowledge of the brain and how it processes memory and makes meaning, and its need for social interaction and appropriate level of stress and challenge
- Rapid societal and technological change: political and economic revolutions that influence what and how learning takes place

The students arriving at school in the 21st century are *digital experts*. Technology has been an integral part of their lives and, for some, a compelling attention-getter. Students today are wired differently because of daily exposure to technology. In *Teaching Digital Natives*, Marc Prensky (2010) explains that students want to live in today's world using today's tools.

Figure 1.2 shows three distinct categories and skills within each that should be embedded in curriculum.

Along with all these issues is the fact that we are teaching students not for our lifetime but for the future, and teachers using the CCSS are also integrating skills for the 21st century:

- Thinking critically and making judgments
- Solving complex, multidisciplinary, open-ended problems
- Creativity and entrepreneurial thinking
- Communicating and collaborating
- Making innovative use of knowledge, information, and opportunities
- Taking charge of financial, health, and civic responsibilities

Schools are expected to build in opportunities within the curriculum for students to practice and develop these skills. However, the balancing act involves dealing

Figure 1.2 Categories and Related Skills to Embed in the Curriculum

Learning and Innovation The 4 Cs	Digital Literacy	Career and Life
• Critical thinking and problem solving • Creativity and innovation • Communication • Collaboration	• Information literacy • Media literacy • Information and communication technology literacy	• Flexibility and adaptability • Initiative and self-direction • Social and cross-cultural interaction • Productivity and accountability

with the CCSS and the reality that classrooms contain diverse, heterogeneous groups of learners. Learners with different cultural backgrounds, experiences, interests, learning preferences, and multiple intelligences are the norm.

Students do not all learn the same thing in the same way on the same day. As educators in classrooms, we need to consider each child in the learning community, based on his or her needs, readiness, preferences, and interests.

We live and work in a global society of high accountability. The legislative notion that any educator would willingly "leave a child behind" is insulting to most educators who view their chosen profession as a mission rather than as a job.

For many decades, educators used a bell curve to rank students. They didn't expect everyone to succeed. It was more the norm to "teach, test, and hope for the best." Today, however, we do expect that all students will learn to their full potential and that all teachers will find a way to enable each individual to be successful. Dr. R. L. Canady, of the University of Virginia, has shared that there are three groups of students in classrooms:

- A group of 25% to 37% of students learn "in spite of us." Those are the students who come ready, willing, and prepared to play the school game in order to succeed. These learners see education as a means to an end, do the work as assigned regardless of preferences, and have the support of significant others in their lives.
- A group of 15% to 25% of students are identified as having some exceptionality and receive additional resources.
- A large group of about 37% to 50% learn because of the teacher's skills and efforts and because of appropriate instruction and assessment aligned with CCSS targeted standards.

Through differentiation, we give all these students the opportunity to learn to their full potential. Throughout this book, we explore the elements needed in the differentiated classroom to engage students and to facilitate learning in order to increase the chances that all learners will succeed. Figure 1.3 organizes these elements in categories, listing tools and strategies that build an inclusive, nurturing classroom and allow teachers to design learning to honor the diversity of the learning population.

Figure 1.3 Tools and Strategies for Designing Inclusive Differentiated Classrooms for Diverse Learners

Climate	Knowing the Learner	Assessing the Learner	Adjustable Assignments	Instructional Strategies	Curriculum Approaches
Safe **Nurturing** **Encourages Risk Taking** **Multisensory** **Stimulating** **Complex** **Challenging** **Collaborative** **Team and Class Building** **Norms** **Mindset**	Learning Profiles Learning Preferences Sweet Spot Dunn & Dunn Gregorc Silver/Strong/Hanson **Multiple Intelligences** Using observation checklists, inventories, logs, and journals to become more aware of how students learn Cultural Gender Pop culture	**Before** Preassessment Formal Pretest Journaling Informal Squaring off Boxing Graffiti facts **During** Formative Formal Journaling/Portfolios Teacher-made tests Checklists/Rubrics Informal Thumb it Fist of five Face the fact **After** Formal Summative Posttest Portfolio/Conferences Reflections Informal Talking topics Conversation Circles Donut	**Compacting** Gifted **TAPS** Total Group Lecturette Presentation Demonstration Jigsaw Video Field trip Guest speaker Text Alone Interest Personalized Multiple intelligences Paired Random Interest Task Small Groups Heterogeneous Homogeneous Task Oriented Constructed Random Interest	**Edu-neuroscience and Differentiation** **Brain facts** Memory model Elaborative rehearsal Focus activities Graphic organizers Compare & contrast Webbing Metaphorical thinking Cooperative group learning Jigsaw Questioning Cubing Role-play Technology	Centers Projects Choice Boards Problem-Based Learning Inquiry Models Contracts

PLANNING FOR DIFFERENTIATED INSTRUCTION

A planning model (see Figure 1.4) can be used to help teachers make decisions about differentiated instruction and assessment. Each phase of the planning model will be explained. Throughout this book, the strategies are clarified using examples.

1. Establish what needs to be taught. First, consider the CCSS, anchor standards and English language arts standards across the content areas, benchmarks, essential questions, or expectations to be taught. It should be clear what the students should know, be able to do, or be like after the learning experience. Determine which formative assessment strategies will be used to collect data (e.g., logs, checklists, journals, observations, portfolios, rubrics). Also create an appropriate final assessment that clearly shows whether students have achieved the CCSS. **Essential questions** may be developed that will be visible and posted throughout the unit so that students can consider the questions as they work on tasks.

2. Identify the **content,** including knowledge, understandings, and essential skills.

3. **Activate.** Determine what students know and what they need to learn next. This accesses prior knowledge that has been stored in the brain's long-term memory. This formative pre-assessment may be done 1 to 3 weeks prior to the unit to allow plenty of time for planning learning activities, grouping students, and raising anticipation and excitement about the new topic. "Emotional hooks" can be used to engage students and to capture their attention as the brain responds to challenge, novelty, and unique experiences.

A strong pre-assessment determines what the students know. The pre-assessment is sometimes formal and sometimes informal. It is essential to select an assessment tool that best shows students' prior knowledge, background experience, and attitudes and preferences toward the information. The interpretation of the gathered data needs to drive planning in order to provide quality learning opportunities.

4. **Acquire.** Decide what new knowledge and skills students need to learn and how they will acquire them to the level of understanding. Also decide whether the acquisition will take place in a total-group setting or in small groups and whether it will be based on readiness or interest.

Now it is time to lay out the plan. Determine how the information can best be taught to this particular group or groups of students. Weed through the resources available, and find the materials that will best meet the needs of these students. Focus on quality materials, and remember that what works for one group does not always work for another group. Also create the formative assessments to be used throughout the learning as benchmarks on the way to success. These will check for understanding or skill level and provide data for next instructional steps. These may not always be graded but will inform instruction.

5. **Apply and Adjust.** Students need the opportunity to practice and become actively engaged with the new learning in order to understand and retain it. Remember, of course, to build in opportunities to use both academic and domain-specific vocabulary and a variety of levels of thinking and complexity as noted in the CCSS. Determine how the students will be grouped and what tasks will be assigned to challenge them at the appropriate levels. The brain needs multiple rehearsals to strengthen the dendritic connections in the neocortex so that new learning is

Figure 1.4 The Six-Step Planning Model for Differentiated Learning: Template

Planning for Differentiated Learning	
1. CORE STANDARDS: What should students know and be able to do?	Assessment tools for data collection: (logs, checklists, journals, agendas, observations, portfolios, rubrics, contracts)
Essential Questions:	
2. CONTENT: (concepts, vocabulary, facts) SKILLS:	
3. ACTIVATE: Focus Activity: Pre-assessment strategy Pre-assessment Prior knowledge & engaging the learners	• Quiz, test • Surveys • K-W-L • Journals • Arm gauge • Give me • Brainstorm • Concept formation • Thumb it
4. ACQUIRE: Total group or small groups	• Lecturette • Presentation • Demonstration • Jigsaw • Video • Field trip • Guest speaker • Text
5. Grouping Decisions: (TAPS, random, heterogeneous, homogeneous, interest, task, constructed) APPLY FORMative assessments ADJUST	• Learning centers • Projects • Contracts • Compact/Enrichment • Problem based • Inquiry • Research • Independent study
6. Summative ASSESSMENT Diversity Honored (learning styles, multiple intelligences, personal interest, etc.)	• Quiz, test • Performance • Products • Presentation • Demonstration • Log, journal • Checklist • Portfolio • Rubric • Metacognition

transferred to long-term memory. This can determine the need for interventions to be addressed and which students need to revisit missed segments in the foundation required to learn the new information. Also, the learners who already know the information may need challenging assignments to enhance their knowledge.

6. **Assess.** Have the students demonstrate their knowledge. Consider providing choices for doing so. Select a quality formative assessment tool that will provide the best evidence of the information mastered, needing planned interventions, and the parts that need to be spiraled back through at a later date. Determine what will be the most effective summative assessment and how will it be graded.

All these decisions are made with the intention of honoring the diversity of the students' learning preferences, multiple intelligences, and personal interests. This instructional plan also addresses and honors the differences in the knowledge base and experiences of each learner as students move toward meeting the CCSS.

Remember, the implementation theme of "one size doesn't fit all" proves that there is a need to differentiate instruction. So let's get started exploring the facets of differentiating instruction and offering our students diverse opportunities to succeed.

Chapter 1
Reflections

1. In interest groups or alone, brainstorm ways you meet the individual needs of students. After compiling the list, post it and title it "Ways to Differentiate Instruction."

2. Differentiated instruction is like _____ (select a noun) because _____ (list the many ways the two are alike). Illustrate, share, and post.

3. In groups of four, jigsaw the four ways to differentiate (a) content, (b) formative assessment, (c) performance assessment, and (d) instructional strategies. Each team member reads the section in the book on his or her assigned topic, takes notes, and adds how he or she currently differentiates in this area. Then each participant shares his or her gathered information while the other group members take notes.

4. Use Figure 1.3 to take a personal inventory of your current use of differentiated instruction. Place a star by the areas that you are implementing. Place a check by the areas that you have used but not very often. Place an X by the areas that you have not used.

2

Creating a Climate for Learning

CLASSROOMS EVERYWHERE OFFER A DIVERSITY OF FACES AND shapes and sizes, but underneath the diversity, there are fundamental elements that all learners need in order to succeed and to feel positive about their experiences in school.

WHAT DO LEARNERS NEED TO SUCCEED?

For students to succeed, they need to believe that they can learn and that what they are learning is useful, relevant, and meaningful for them. They need to know that they belong in the classroom and that they are responsible for their own learning and behavior. This develops a self-directed learner who is confident in making the information his or her own. This instills *self-efficacy*, which means believing in oneself. In *Education on the Edge of Possibility*, Renate and Geoffrey Caine (1997) state,

> Teachers' beliefs in and about human potential and in the ability of all children to learn and achieve are critical. These aspects of the teachers' mental models have a profound impact on the learning climate and learner states of mind that teachers create. Teachers need to understand students' feelings and attitudes will be involved and will profoundly influence student learning. (p. 124)

Effective teachers believe that all students can learn and be successful. Effective teachers consciously create a climate in which all students feel included. Effective teachers believe that there is potential in each learner and commit to finding the key that will unlock that potential.

Teacher Mindsets

Carol Dweck (2006) is a researcher as well as a psychology professor at Stanford, and her book *Mindset: The New Psychology of Success* discusses motivation and intelligence. She explains that some people have different beliefs about intelligence and ability. Dweck believes that people are on different places on the continuum between *fixed* and *growth* based on their view of intelligence, effort, and success. You are said to have a growth mindset if you believe success and abilities come from hard work and you "keep on keeping on" despite challenges and disappointments. People with a growth mindset believe in multiple opportunities to be successful. Those with a fixed mindset, on the other hand, believe that intelligence is an innate ability that has limits. Failure for them reinforces their view of limitations, and they are not motivated to continue working at the task. Effective teachers have positive mindsets that guide their behavior in the classroom and their interactions with students (R. Brooks & Goldstein, 2008).

A teacher's mindset influences students' mindsets. Everything we say and do should give the message of possibility and influence the students' perception of their capabilities while fostering optimism and tenacity. Both students' successes and efforts should receive feedback and response giving them the message that we all can continue to get better. The phrases in Figure 2.1 may be used to respond to students' successes and earnest attempts. These both validate achievement and encourage student perseverance.

CLASSROOM CULTURE AND LEARNING COMMUNITIES

Culture is often referred to as "the way we do things around here." People who live and work in a culture sometimes can't explain or describe it, but they can certainly

Figure 2.1 Encouraging Feedback Prompts to Use With Students

Feedback for Success	Feedback to Encourage
Great effort	You're on the way
Well done	Keep practicing
You did it	Keep trying
Your practice paid off	You'll get it
I knew you could do it	One more time and you'll have it
You've hit the mark	I know you can
Aren't you proud of yourself	You will
You've got that down pat	Don't stop now
Nice going	You're on the right track
I never doubted you	Keep on trucking
	Try, try, try again

sense it. Culture may not necessarily be conveyed only through words, but also through actions. Sometimes what we do screams so loudly that we can't hear what is being said. In the words of DePorter, Reardon, and Singer-Nourie (1998), in their book *Quantum Teaching*, "everything speaks, everything always." They caution teachers that what they do, say, and allude to has an effect on learners and their perceptions of success. According to Gregory and Parry (2006),

> as far as the brain is concerned, actions speak louder than words. Everything that happens in the classroom is monitored by three parts of the brain, two of which have no spoken language but are very adept at reading body language and tone of voice. Every gesture, every inflection, and every invasion of personal space is monitored by the limbic system and evaluated in terms of its threat potential. These skills allowed our ancestors to survive and they are still alive and well in all of us. (p. 13)

Because the brain is a *parallel processor,* it absorbs information on conscious and unconscious levels. The brain constantly performs many functions at the same time (Ornstein & Thompson, 1984). It therefore can manage to process thoughts, emotions, and perceptions simultaneously.

The brain is also a parallel processor in that it facilitates learning by involving both focused attention and peripheral perception. O'Keefe and Nadel (1978) state that the brain responds to the entire sensory context in which learning takes place. *Peripheral stimuli* include everything in the classroom, from the drab or colorful walls to subtle clues, such as a look or gesture, that convey meaning and are interpreted by the brain. All sounds and visual signals are full of complex messages. A sarcastic remark can speak volumes to a sensitive learner, and a gesture can convey far more than the spoken word.

In his work with the Mid-continent Research for Education and Learning group and with Dimensions of Learning, Robert Marzano (1992) examined the climate for learning. Jay McTighe (1990) did as well, with the Maryland State Department of Education:

> Closely related to teachers' behavior is the development of a classroom climate conducive to good thinking. . . . [S]tudents cannot think well in a harsh, threatening situation or even in a subtly intimidating environment where group pressure makes independent thinking unlikely. Teachers can make their classrooms more thoughtful places by demonstrating in their actions that they welcome originality and differences of opinion.

Noted researcher Deborah Rozman (1998) remarks that "the neural information the heart sends to the brain can either facilitate or inhibit cortical function, affecting perception, emotional response, learning, and decision making." The heartbeat of another person is perceivable within 3 to 4 feet, because of the electromagnetic field that it projects. The heartbeat of one person registers in the brainwaves of another person. There are intuitive or gut feelings that are picked up by neurons throughout the body. It has often been said, "People need to know you care before they care what you know." And old adages become just that because they are usually true.

As part of his choice theory of motivation, William Glasser (1990, 1998) cites five equally important needs:

- The need to survive and reproduce
- The need to belong and love
- The need to have some power
- The need to have freedom
- The need to have fun

This is also evident in Abraham Maslow's (1968) well-known hierarchy of needs, which includes the following, beginning with the most basic:

- Physiological needs: food, water, air, shelter
- Safety needs: security, freedom from fear, order
- Belongingness and love: friends, spouse, children
- Self-esteem: self-respect, achievement, reputation
- Self-actualization: becoming what the individual has the potential to become

Human beings generally move up the hierarchy from basic to complex needs. As each need has been met, it becomes less of a motivator as the person focuses on the next level.

As we examine motivators, we need to remember that basic needs have to be met first for students. We recognize that all humans have a very strong need to be liked and included. Classrooms everywhere must foster an inclusionary climate. It is essential that students bond with one another and with the teacher to form a positive learning community. Dr. Robert Sapolsky (1998), professor of biological sciences and neuroscience at Stanford University, states that we can minimize the impact of stress by building a supportive environment:

Put an infant primate through something unpleasant: it gets a stress-response. Put it through the same stressor while in a room full of other primates and . . . it depends. If those primates are strangers, the stress-response gets worse. But if they are friends, the stress-response is decreased. Social support networks—it helps to have a shoulder to cry on, a hand to hold, an ear to listen to you, someone to cradle you and to tell you it will be okay. (p. 215)

People need people. The brain is wired to belong. "From a biological standpoint, people deprived of the human moment in their day to day . . . dealings are losing brain cells—literally—while those who cultivate the human moment are growing them" (Hallowell, 2011, p. 9).

Without love and connections we have "atrophy of the limbic system." (Gregory, 2012)

Some teachers work with their students to cooperatively develop classroom *agreements* (Gibbs, 1995), *trust statements* (Harmin, 1994), or "rules to live by" to help students feel that they have a voice in the running of the classroom. These rules also help students become more emotionally intelligent and responsible learners. Students in small groups generate statements that they believe the class should live by, for example, "Everyone's ideas count." After the groups share their statements, the class combines, deletes, or adds sentences until consensus is reached and students feel comfortable and can support these rules to live by, which may include the following:

- There is no wrong opinion.
- No put-downs or sarcasm here.
- Everyone must be heard.
- Mistakes are learning points.

If these statements are posted for all students to see and reflect on, students will monitor and honor the rules that they have created.

We also recognize that learning communities foster links between heart and mind. Driscoll (1994) asks us to consider the following:

> Community is the entity in which individuals derive meaning. It is not so much characterized by shared space as it is by shared meanings. Community in this view is not a mere artifact of people living (or working or studying) in the same place, but is rather a rich source of living tradition. (p. 3)

In today's classroom, learners from many cultures and backgrounds form the classroom community. Teachers need to learn as much as possible about the cultures that are represented in order to be able to understand and reach the students. Some students do not know the native language of the classroom, so it is up to the teacher and the other students to help these students communicate with them and learn the language as soon as possible. The teacher is a role model for students to learn the customs and expectation of the new classroom. Each learner must know that he or she is an important contributing member of the classroom.

EMOTIONS AND LEARNING

Students living in fear cannot learn. Students will not attend to learning if their major concern is safety. The higher the level of stress, the less access to higher levels of thinking and the greater the feeling of flight or fight, a basic survival response. So in classrooms we need to challenge students in ways appropriate to their skill levels without overstressing them. Some students may already be so stressed from difficult situations in their personal lives that they are unable to fully attend to lessons, as they are on high alert (Gregory & Parry, 2006).

Safety in classrooms means intellectual as well as physical safety. During stress, the emotional centers of the brain take control of cognitive functioning; thus the rational, thinking part of the brain is not as efficient, and this can cause learning to be impeded. If students are living daily with the threat of being ridiculed or bullied, they cannot give their full attention to learning. Students who are challenged beyond their skill levels are more concerned about being embarrassed or laughed at than about the quest for learning. They will not be motivated to attempt the challenge if they aren't able to imagine or perceive success.

In classrooms where the teacher does not adjust the learning to the students' levels of readiness and teaches only to the "middle," some students will be bored from lack of challenge, and others may be placed under undue stress from too great a challenge. Thus, teachers need to consider where their learners are in relation to the learning goal and plan learning experiences just beyond the skill level of each student.

All students are more likely to be engaged in the learning, rise to the challenge, and have a sense of self-confidence as they approach the task if they feel that they have a chance to succeed. Thus, once the teacher has considered their levels of readiness, students can often be grouped and experiences designed to accommodate the learners at their levels of understanding.

Teachers need to consider the degree of complexity of learning tasks so that they will be challenging but not overwhelming. This establishes the state of *flow* (Csikszentmihalyi, 1990), the condition that exists when learners are so engaged, excited about learning, challenged, and receiving appropriate feedback that they are oblivious to anything else. Students are at their most productive and most creative in this state:

> People seem to concentrate best when the demands on them are a bit greater than usual, and they are able to give more than usual. If there is too little demand on them, people are bored. If there is too much for them to handle, they get anxious. Flow occurs in that delicate zone between boredom and anxiety. (Goleman, 1992, as cited in Csikszentmihalyi, 1990, p. 4)

Renate Caine, a well-known pioneer in the field of brain-based education, proposes that there are three basic elements to brain/mind learning and teaching:

- Emotional climate and relationship or relaxed alertness
- Instruction or immersion in complex experience
- Consolidation of learning or active processing

Emotional climate and relationships are important in producing what Kohn (1993) refers to as "relaxed alertness":

> All the methodologies that are used to orchestrate the learning context influence the state of relaxed alertness. It is particularly important for educators to understand the effect of rewards and punishments on student states of mind. Research shows most applications of reward and punishment in the behavioral mode inhibit creativity, interfere with intrinsic motivation, and reduce the likelihood of meaningful learning. (as cited in R. N. Caine & Caine, 1997, p. 123)

Rewards and punishments tend to lessen the chances of self-motivation and an appreciation of learning as its own reward. Here are five practical alternatives to using rewards:

- Eliminating threat
- Creating a strongly positive climate
- Increasing feedback
- Setting goals
- Activating and engaging positive emotions (Jensen, 1998b, p. 68)

It is important, if not imperative, that students feel good, have success, have friends, and celebrate their learning:

> Emotions affect student behavior because they create distinct, mind-body states. A state is a moment composed of a specific posture, breathing rate, and chemical balance in the body. The presence or absence of [brain neurotransmitters such as] norepinephrine, vasopressin, testosterone, serotonin, progesterone, dopamine, and dozens of other chemicals dramatically alters your frame of mind and body. How important are states to us? They are all that we have; they are our feelings, desires, memories, and motivations. (Jensen, 1998b, p. 75)

The emotional environment interacts with instruction and influences how information is consolidated. If undue stress occurs, the high stress/threat response, or automatic reflex response, sabotages connections and thus learning cannot take place. At this point, we are fortunate if even memorization of isolated facts and programmed skills is possible. It is almost impossible for higher-order thinking to take place.

If a student thinks that success isn't possible because the task is too difficult or instructions for a task are ambiguous and not understood, he or she feels uncertain. This causes the learner to form a negative state, and the learner ceases to persevere. Alternately, classrooms that create *eustress*, or a state of flow, create a positive learning environment. Classrooms that embed choices in learning and routines that demonstrate mutual respect are supportive learning environments for students. Attending to routines, patterns, and clear expectations in the classroom lowers anticipation anxiety that is created when students are uneasy about what to expect and the unknown.

EMOTIONAL INTELLIGENCE

Emotional intelligence is a person's ability to use his or her emotions intelligently. It involves maintaining a balance between reason and emotion. Daniel Goleman (1995) organizes emotional intelligence as a set of emotional competencies that occur in five domains: self-awareness, managing emotions, self-motivation, empathy, and social skills. Emotional intelligence, especially the acquisition of social skills, is a key skill for the 21st century.

Self-Awareness

Self-awareness is one's ability to sense and name a feeling when it happens and also to put it into words. Self-aware people can use appropriate strategies to deal with their moods by sharing frustrations with others or seeking support on a bad day. Teachers should encourage students to articulate their feelings and seek and give support. Self-awareness also involves being in touch with feelings, not letting feelings become engulfing, and having strategies to cope with moods. In her book *Molecules of Emotion*, Candace B. Pert (1998) suggests, "Feeling low and sluggish? Take a walk. Feeling anxious and jittery? Run!" (p. 293). We all need to find ways to change and manage our moods once we recognize what they are.

Managing Emotions

Managing emotions is an outcome of recognizing and labeling feelings. It is the ability to calm and soothe during anxious moments or to manage and deal with anger. Using teachable moments (when an inappropriate emotional response has been given), teachers can help students learn problem-solving skills to generate appropriate alternatives to the feelings. Conflict resolution is easier if students have a repertoire of strategies for dealing with conflict when it erupts.

Self-Motivation

Self-motivation consists of competencies such as persistence, setting one's own goals, and delaying gratification. Many students give up very easily when difficulties occur. Students need to feel hopeful even in the face of setback. The state of flow is an integral component of this domain. If students and teachers can create that state of high challenge and low threat, more learning can take place.

Empathy

Empathy is being able to feel for another. Teachers can ask students to "stand in the other person's shoes." That other person may be a classmate in a situation that calls for empathy or a character in fiction or history with whom students can empathize to understand the person's emotions. This allows the students to feel how the character or individual might have felt. Understanding another's point of view or perspective is often a standard targeted in many districts. Feeling for others builds tolerance and understanding.

Social Skills

Social skills are the competencies that one uses to "read" other people and manage emotional interactions. People with high levels of social competencies have the ability to handle relationships well and are able to adapt to a variety of social situations. They are said to have "social polish." Teachers modeling these competencies and labeling them when seen in the classroom show the value of emotional intelligence in personal interactions.

The Emotional Intelligence Chart (see Figure 2.2) lists the five domains of emotional intelligence and gives suggestions for fostering each intelligence and strategies for classroom applications.

SELF-REGULATION

Self-regulation is defined as regulation of the self by the self (Baumeister & Vohs, 2006). Self-regulation is the ability to adapt your mental, emotional, and physiological state to the task at hand. It enables students to control their behavior, get along with others, and attend to learning by being calm and focused. Stuart Shanker, a distinguished researcher at York University, in Canada, suggests that whereas IQ was a predictor of success in the 20th century, self-regulation is more indicative of success in the 21st century (Shanker & Downer, 2012). Genes and temperament influence how well children are able to self-regulate. Without self-regulation, they struggle to cope. And with so much energy wasted on coping, there will be little left to pay attention, control impulses, remember, and learn.

Figure 2.2   Emotional Intelligence Chart

Intelligence	To Foster	Strategies for Application
Self-awareness: One's ability to sense and name a feeling when it happens	Help students discuss their feelings in different situations.	Reflection Logs and journals
Managing emotions: Recognizing and labeling feelings and responding appropriately	Use "teachable moments" to help students learn to manage emotions.	Deep breathing Counting to 10 Taking time out Physical movement
Self-motivation: Competencies such as persistence, goal setting, and delaying gratification	Help students find a niche. Help them to persist in difficult or challenging situations.	Goal setting Persistence strategies Problem solving
Empathy: Ability to feel for another person	Encourage students to "stand in another's shoes." Think about another person's pain.	Modeling empathy Discussing empathic responses to persons studied
Social skills: Competencies that one uses to "read" and manage emotional interactions	Teach social skills explicitly. Have students practice social skills while doing group tasks.	Modeling social skills Using explicit language to describe behaviors, so students can practice the skills

Students are in charge of monitoring and controlling their learning. Cognitive information processing constructs new information or information products. Teachers model the processing of information and problem-solving techniques. The learners then build a toolbox of strategies. Each individual has to select his or her way to learn information and place it in a long-term memory bank. Teachers need to allow time for students to ponder and come up with their own way to learn the information. Another way for students to have control of their learning is for the teacher to provide choices. It is important for students to show what they know to determine the next steps in learning.

Different situations call for their own appropriate behavior, for example, how a student should act at school. These behaviors are taught, explained, and usually have established rules and regulations. It is up to the individual to decide to follow the rules or not. The decision of how to act is within his or her control.

Motivation to learn is an inward desire. It is up to the teacher to plan exciting, memorable learning experiences that capture and stimulate the desire to learn and participate. Self-regulated learning skills do not develop automatically, but once developed these skills will benefit students for lifelong learning. When students have difficulty with self-regulation, they may need to go to a quiet area to work, or they may need some physical movement to reduce the stress and anxiety and then refocus on the task. Therefore, it is worth the time for teachers and parents to help students develop their self-regulatory competencies and encourage them to practice using them in all facets of their lives.

CLASSROOM CLIMATE

Learning Atmosphere

In a differentiated classroom, students feel safe and secure enough to take risks and express their understanding or lack of understanding. Many times, the students considered academically gifted feel that they are expected to know all the information. Often these learners pretend to have all the answers in response to the expectations of others. This can cause stress and interfere with learning. A disappointed look or comment can keep gifted students from expressing a lack of understanding. These students, like all other students, should feel secure in the classroom even when they don't have all the answers.

Learners who are considered to be at risk or low achieving often live up to the expectations of the label. Giving students a look of surprise when they "get it" shows that they are not expected to get it! Often this puts a cap on potential. When the "aha" moment occurs, the student needs to go tell a peer how the problem was solved and reveal his or her thinking process. That makes for motivated peer tutors, and each time the learner explains his or her thinking, the information is being rehearsed again and the connections in the brain are strengthened. This respects the student's accomplishment with a needed celebration.

In a differentiated classroom, the emphasis is on knowledge base and experience rather than IQ and ability. Each student is respected. Learners know that learning is a process and everyone learns differently. Learning includes weeding out what students know with effective pre-assessments and ongoing formative assessments to determine what students need next. Teachers should foster a growth mindset in students by helping them understand that practice makes perfect, some of us need more practice to understand and develop skills, and that's okay. We can all get better if we persist. This policy establishes a different mindset of being able to admit mistakes, accept lack of understanding, and celebrate successes and growth in an individual's knowledge base. Teachers' verbal or written feedback to students also should reinforce effort and persistence, not just praise or criticism. "Good job. You really worked hard on finishing that. I liked the way you kept searching until you found the information you needed." Each moment of successful improvement makes a positive change for a lifetime.

Physical and Emotional Atmosphere

The climate is influenced by the physical attributes of the classroom. Things such as appropriate lighting, cleanliness, orderliness, and displays of students' work contribute to a positive atmosphere. Plentiful and appropriate resources are necessary to facilitate student success. There could be computers and materials that allow for hands-on manipulation. There should also be opportunities for social interaction and intellectual growth.

Enriched environments are created not only by materials but also by the complexity and variety of tasks, challenges, and feedback. Engaging materials and activities help to develop *dendritic growth,* the neural connections that are facilitated by experiences and stimulation.

The message is clear: Although the brain possesses a relatively constant macro structural organization, the ever-changing cerebral cortex, with its complex micro architecture of unknown potential, is powerfully shaped by experiences before birth, during youth and, in fact, throughout life. It is essential to note that enrichment effects on the brain have consequences on behavior. Parents, educators, policy makers, and individuals can all benefit from such knowledge. (Diamond, 2001)

Use of the Arts

Another component of enhancing classroom climate may be the inclusion of different genres and media from the art classroom, which can assist learners in gaining understanding of difficult material. It has been said that a picture is worth a thousand words, and in fact, the brain processes visuals up to 60,000 times faster than words. This is true because a picture makes unknown information come alive for the learner. When the textbook or the teacher refers to an unfamiliar noun, a student can go to the computer and find an informative picture to gain a better understanding of the word. Pictures let learners see whatever they are reading and hearing. Students can make sketches or drawings to create meaning for unfamiliar words. These visuals create personal ownership for students. Folding booklets and graphic organizers are effective differentiated instructional strategies to use across the content areas to teach and assist learners in organizing their ideas and recording needed information.

Classroom climate can also be enhanced with the inclusion of music. Researchers at Strathclyde University have discovered that brainpower soars when students listen to stimulating pop tunes, and they advise that playing the latest hits in classrooms may actually increase student achievement. This study, by Dr. Brian Boyd and Katrina Bowes (*The Brain in the News,* Dana Press, 2001), researched the effects of music after learning about studies in Russia. The researchers discovered that medical patients who listened to music recovered faster. In contrast to the belief that only classical music calms the learner, they found that modern music with the same tempo as classical (60 beats per minute) has the same effect and makes the mind more receptive to learning. This music can actually help the brain retain information.

Many teachers who have tried using pop music report higher levels of concentration by their students. Pop music triggers the autonomic nervous system, and we respond by feeling good and tapping our feet to the music. The pupils of the eyes dilate, and endorphin levels and energy rise. Teachers often say that students will learn more in a class if they are enjoying the experience, and music can set the stage for learning. Students will link a known routine with a piece of music and thus be ready for what is to follow. The music can be playful and related to the lesson, for example, playing Marvin Gaye's "I Heard It Through the Grapevine" while students are estimating the number of raisins in a small, lunch-size box. Or the music can appeal to the emotions and create a mood, as when listening to "When Johnny Comes Marching Home Again" at the beginning of a discussion of World War I or "War," by Bruce Springsteen, in relation to the study of the Vietnam War.

Music energizes people and masks "dead air" when there is a dip in students' energy level. Mozart's music or Baroque music can soothe and calm as well (Campbell, 1998).

Today students walk around with earbuds in, listening to music while completing difficult tasks. Some individuals learn and work more efficiently while listening to music. For others, music interferes with concentration on an assigned task. If students are allowed to play personal music during class, establish some rules. Consider the following guidelines:

- Allow earbud use at times determined by the teacher.
- Give students a choice of listening or not listening to music.
- Obtain teacher approval of the music selections or sources.

Play music as hooks or closures to introduce a segment of learning, to set a mood or tone, and to create a jiving transition. Enjoy the arts as you integrate them across the curriculum.

Laughter and Celebrating Learning

Laughter is another tool to use in classrooms. It punctuates learning by releasing neurochemical transmitters called *endorphins,* and it is said to be the shortest distance between two people. Laughter even helps the immune system increase the number of type T leukocytes (T cells) in the blood. T cells combat damage and infection, and some researchers have even dubbed them "happiness cells" (Cardoso, 2000). It makes sense to include humor and laughter and to celebrate learning in the classroom. Teachers can encourage students to applaud one another and cheer for each other's successes. Using energizing cheers (Burke, 1993; DePorter et al., 1998), students can give rounds of applause, high fives, and other cheers that they can often create for themselves. These cheers also include actions to supplement the aural responses. Kinesthetic actions help energize students by sending more oxygen and glucose to the brain and often result in fun and laughter to raise endorphins.

Celebrating learning is important for students of all ages. A simple way to celebrate any classroom success is to lead an energizing cheer. When an individual or small group has a "lightbulb moment" or presents what has been learned, give a cheer. Besides the emotional boost, these cheers provide a physical boost to the brain. The physical actions send oxygen and glucose to the brain.

The following are some examples of cheers and activities that energize and celebrate. Add your own physical movements to punctuate the cheer:

- Make a fist and raise arm in the air. Bring down and yell, "Yes!"
- *Triple Yes!!!* Repeat the "Yes" three time with the above hand motion.
- *Oh, Yes!* Make a circle over the head with both arms and say, "Oh!" Then bring the hand in a balled fist down from the top to make the cheering Yes!
- *Ketchup Clap.* Make a fist with one hand, and hit on top of the fist with the other hand. It is like getting ketchup to come out of the bottle.
- *Fish Clap.* Open one hand. Flap the other hand back and forth in the palm of the open hand.
- *Table Rap Clap.* Rap on the table while saying, "Table rap." Then clap hands while saying, "Clap."
- *Happy Clam Clap.* Make a smiley face with hands across mouth while saying, "Happy." Then hit fingers against the thumb like a clam opening and shutting them and say, "Clam clap."
- *Wah hoo!* Yell "Wah hoo!" while bringing arm across the front of the body and raising it high in the air.
- *Awesome.* Put hands above the head and bow down while saying, "Awesome."
- *Wow.* With three fingers on each hand, make a W on each side of the mouth. Open mouth to form the O and say, "Wow!"
- *Microwave.* Wave with your little finger.

- *Standing oh!* Stand up and make a circle with arms around your head and say, "Oh!"
- *You did it!* Repeat three times in a rhythmic pattern while moving to the beat.
- *High Five.* Raise up hand and wave.
- *Excellent Guitar.* Pretend to strum a guitar and strum while saying, "Excellent."
- *Round of Applause.* Make a circle of claps.
- *You are great and getting greater!* Chant the cheer with no motions.

Each learner in the classroom is very different, and everyone needs to feel safe and comfortable. In classrooms, climate and atmosphere play an important part in the learning process. Anything teachers can do to create a risk-free supportive environment where students can feel safe and where they can thrive needs to be considered and implemented. Building a community of learners who care for and support one another is essential in a differentiated classroom. Students who know and respect each other are more tolerant of differences and more comfortable when tasks are different. Even though "one size doesn't fit all," learners require all these conditions to succeed.

Chapter 2 Reflections

Taking the time to examine some of the concepts in this chapter is something you could do with your professional learning community. It may prompt discussion and reflection on classroom climate and why it is so crucial to learning.

1. How would you describe your classroom climate? What does it look like, sound like, feel like?

2. What goals can you set for improving climate as a team and as an individual?

3. How do you encourage team building throughout the year?

4. What do you do to create a classroom atmosphere in which students can take intellectual risks?

5. How do you create intellectual safety and prohibit ridicule, put-downs, and other negative responses in your classroom?

6. How much wait time do you allow for thinking and answering questions?

7. What steps will you take to create an inclusive atmosphere in which students feel safe and included?

8. How can you foster relaxed alertness?

9. How can you create flow?

3

Knowing the Learner

W E LOOK IN CLASSROOMS AT SCHOOLS AND OBSERVE THE variety of students in all different shapes and sizes. They all look different, and they are. As with clothing, their sizes vary, and each wearer has individual preferences for style, color, and occasion.

Could we buy clothing for children we didn't know? We would need to find out about them as individuals, ask about their likes and dislikes, preferences for color and style, and of course their sizes. We would never consider buying just anything and hope that it would fit and appeal to the recipient. So in classrooms, we need to know the learners so that we can make sure the curriculum fits.

Many teachers have spent summers writing and designing curricula that focus on standards and are intended to engage learners. But when they met the students in the classroom, the program didn't fit their needs, interests, preferences, readiness levels, or appeal to them (or, it might be said, "They sent the wrong students"). It is important to look at the reality in our classrooms, recognizing that each learner is unique and that what would engage or intrigue one learner wouldn't have the slightest chance of capturing the attention of another student. Part of the reason for this situation is that students have "designer brains," as noted cognitive researcher Robert Sylwester (1995) points out. That is to say, their brains differ as much as their fingerprints and faces do. Over the years, a variety of experts have shared with educators the notion of student learning styles and the fact that we all learn in different ways, process information differently, and have distinct preferences about where, when, and how we learn.

LEARNING PROFILES

A learning profile is a compilation of data to identify and share the ways in which each student learns. It includes but is not limited to how the student perceives the world, accesses information, processes information, learns, thinks, and remembers.

There is limited research in the field of neuroscience that supports the idea that individuals learn in different ways by using different neural pathways when we undertake similar tasks. However, cognitive psychologists seem to perpetuate the notion that learners have different styles that dominate their learning.

John Geake (2009) suggests that most brains follow a normal developmental trajectory; each is also idiosyncratic in its strengths and weaknesses for learning particular types of information.

The Sweet Spot

In the sports realm the term *sweet spot* is the point or area on a bat, club, or racket at which it makes most effective contact with the ball or a place where a combination of factors results in a maximum response for a given amount of effort. Therefore, as teachers it is imperative that we find the sweet spot that will connect the learner with the new learning in the most relevant, efficient way, resulting in a "home run" for learning. Gregory and Kaufeldt (2012) suggest that to find the student's sweet spot we consider what will garner the learner's attention and interest, building on prior avenues of success and providing learning experiences that will create joy and safety. Figure 3.1 shows how these elements intersect to identify the sweet spot. Discovering and attending to the student's sweet spot will hopefully maximize the learning experiences and create student success.

Figure 3.1   Considering the Learner's Sweet Spot

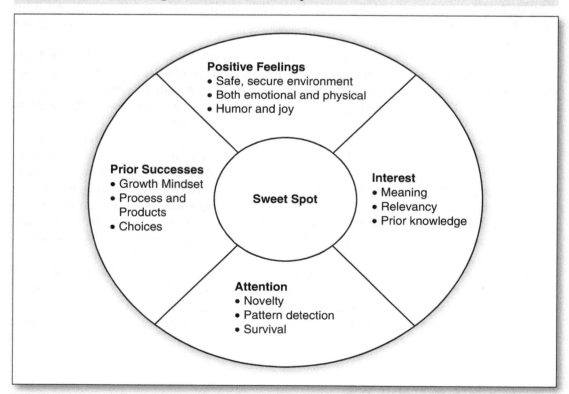

To identify the sweet spot and develop learning profiles, teachers may take different approaches. Here are four ways profiles may be created:

Formally: Create and use surveys and inventories.

Informally: Make observations and anecdotal notes about students' choices, preferences, and excitement or frustration related to a task.

Trial and Error: Cast a broad net of opportunities so that all students can find their niche based on their preferences.

Metacognitive: Provide strategies so that students can reflect on their choices, feelings, and successes as well as set goals. Students need multiple opportunities for reflection and metacognition (thinking about their thinking) related to their work. What went well, what needs improvement, and what goal to set are all things to reflect on in order to persist and be successful.

Students need to know that

- *effort* and
- *perseverance* lead to
- *success.*

This will also foster a *growth mindset*.

Learning profiles are worth creating especially for students who are hard to engage and motivate. The more teachers knows about students, the better they can respond to their preferences. A caution would be to not create a learning profile if you are not going to respond to what you find out about the learner. Remember, profiles evolve over time and are a dynamic tool. They may even be passed on to the next teacher to give him or her a "heads up" and save time in getting to know the learners and their needs. Also, don't leave the students out of the loop; the more students know about the ways they learn and can act on them, the more effective their learning will be (Donavan & Bransford, 2005).

There are seven categories that can be considered to capture student preferences:

1. *Differences in learning:* These seem to be evident and categorized by multiple researchers as well as psychologists who help the teacher and student know how they can best access and process information and deal with their approach and preferences to the learning.

2. *Differences in sensory-based learning:* Students have preferences based on how they best process information through their senses. Sensory source preferences include auditory, visual, and tactile/kinesthetic. Teachers who provide a multisensory classroom will be a step ahead and will satisfy more learners by offering a variety of modes of processing and learning.

3. *Differences in thinking:* A theory of thinking styles is based on two variables: the way we view the world in an abstract or concrete way and the way we order the world in either a sequential or random order.

4. *Differences in multiple intelligences*: Children have various strengths and needs for growth in the areas of multiple intelligences. Howard Gardner (2004, 2006) describes eight intelligences: verbal-linguistic, musical-rhythmic, logical-mathematical, spatial, bodily-kinesthetic, intrapersonal, intrapersonal, and

naturalistic. Existential intelligence is also being explored. Teachers consciously including all intelligences over time will provide students with areas of comfort and areas that might not be as strong, where they will be stretching and developing.

5. *Gender differences:* There are anatomical differences in boys' and girls' brains, and thus they have different needs in the learning process (Gurian, Henley, & Trueman, 2001).

6. *Cultural differences:* All students—regardless of ethnicity—have cultural differences that influence their approach to learning and their needs in the classroom.

7. *Students' interests:* A variety of different exposures and experiences cause students to have different interests.

LEARNING PREFERENCES

How do students access, process, and express information? By viewing different theories on learning styles, personality types, and multiple intelligences, educators can learn about the individual preferences by which they and their students learn and solve problems. As more information about each student's learning preferences, modalities, thinking styles, and multiple intelligences is gathered, it allows teachers to use the knowledge of student strengths as an entry point for instruction and to capture attention.

It is also important for students to increase their knowledge of themselves and for teachers to help students develop metacognitive skills for self-assessment and learning for life. Knowing how one learns is necessary information if one is to learn throughout life. Research on instructional strategies at the Maryland State Department of Education indicates that "teachers who help students develop and internalize metacognitive strategies through direct instruction, modeling, and practice promote learning because the effective use of such strategies is one of the primary differences between more and less able learners" (McTighe, 1990).

Sensory-Based Preferences

One learning preferences model, developed by Rita Dunn and Ken Dunn (1987), classifies learning styles as *auditory, visual,* and *kinesthetic:*

- **Auditory Learners** absorb spoken and heard material easily and like to be involved in aural questioning rather than reading materials. They prefer listening to lectures, stories, and songs, and they enjoy variation, such as voice inflection and intonational pitch. They like to discuss and use opportunities to talk about their learning with other students.
- **Visual Learners** learn best from information that they see or read. They like illustrations, pictures, and diagrams. Graphic organizers are useful tools for them to construct meaning visually. Color has an impact on their learning.

- **Tactile/Kinesthetic Learners** learn best by doing and moving, handling materials, writing, drawing, by becoming physically involved in learning activities that are meaningful and relevant in their lives. They enjoy role-playing and simulations and creating models. They appreciate the freedom and opportunity to move about the classroom.

So What Should We Do About That?

It is important for teachers to be aware of the different modalities and provide adequate activities that tap into each of them during the school day.

The more teachers can involve all modalities and learning styles, the more chances they have of engaging learners in using their whole brains and of achieving the Common Core State Standards that have been incorporated into the lesson and unit of study. Rather than trying to categorize students, it would be preferable to provide a wide range of learning activities that consider and respond to each style (see Figure 3.2).

Examine Lesson Plans for Multiple Ways of Processing Information

Is there opportunity for auditory learners to listen, speak, and discuss?

Is the room equipped with audio headsets to provide time for individual students to access audiotapes, CDs, and DVDs?

Do visual learners get information from reading, observing, and viewing?

Is the room visually appealing, with charts, diagrams, pictures, and student representation for the visual learners?

Do tactile learners get a chance to examine, manipulate, and handle materials and models?

Is there ample opportunity for kinesthetic learners to move about as they need or choose to?

Do you build in role-playing and simulations that deepen understanding and satisfy the tactile/kinesthetic learners?

Variety in the classroom satisfies more learners and engages more areas of the brain, thus causing greater learning and retention. It has been said that we learn

10% of what we read,

20% of what we hear,

30% of what we see,

50% of what we see and hear,

70% of what is discussed with others,

80% of what we experience personally, and

95% of what we teach to someone else. (Ekwall & Shanker, 1988)

Figure 3.2   Learning Preferences: Learning Is Affected by Such Factors as Time of Day and Environment

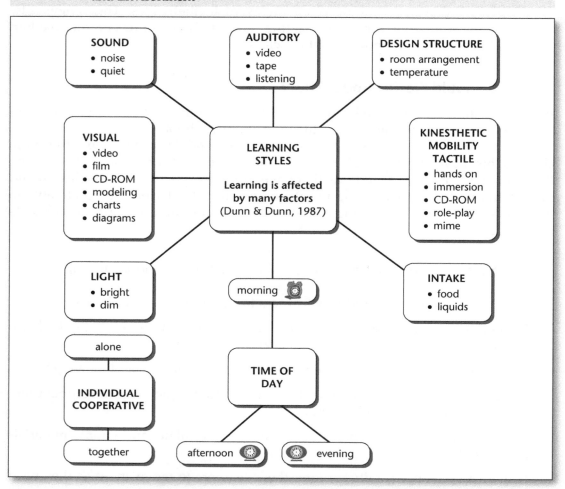

We are not suggesting that we don't read or just listen. We should incorporate all these learning opportunities into classroom experiences so all may be successful and rehearse in a variety of ways, thus aligning with a variety of student learning preferences. They also allow for the inclusion of complex thinking as suggested in the Common Core State Standards.

Figure 3.3 shows retention rates, thinking levels, instructional strategies, and relationship to learning preferences.

Teachers also need to consider other factors that affect learning styles:

- **Noise level:** Do students prefer noise or quiet?
- **Design structure:** What is the preferred room arrangement? Is the room too hot or cold?
- **Motivation and persistence:** Are students able to engage for long or short periods of time?

Figure 3.3   The Relationship Between Retention and Learning Preferences

People Retain	Knowledge Level	Strategies	Preferences
10% Reading	Remember Understand	Test Internet Books Source materials	Visual Clipboard Microscope
20% Lecture	Remember	Lecturette Presentation Talk Guest speaker	Auditory Clipboard Microscopes
30% Audiovisual	Remember Understand	Overhead SMART board Diagrams PowerPoint Charts Pictures Video/DVD Movie Audiotape/CD	Auditory Visual
50% Demonstration	Remember Understand application	Teacher demonstration Virtual reality Internet Webinars	Auditory Visual
70% Discussion	Remember Understand Analyze Evaluate	Partner sharing Small-group learning Social networking	Auditory Interpersonal Verbal-linguistic Puppy
80% Practice	Remember Understand Analyze Apply Evaluate Create	Practicing skills Hands-on projects Verbal rehearsal Manipulatives Models Centers	Auditory Visual Bodily-kinesthetic Beach balls Clipboard
95% Teaching others	Remember Understand Analyze Apply Evaluate Create	Student demonstrations Presentations Exhibition Small-group learning Oral reports	Auditory Verbal-linguistics Interpersonal Puppy Clipboard Microscope Beach ball

Source: Gregory, G. H. (2005). *Differentiating Instruction With Style.* Thousand Oaks, CA: Corwin Press.

- **Responsibility:** Are they fairly independent and self-directed, or do they need a lot of guidance?
- **Structure:** Do they prefer to have more flexibility, or do they need detailed structure?
- **Individual/peer:** Do they like to work with others, or do they prefer to learn alone?

Teachers also can use a learning inventory (see Figure 3.4) to get more data about learners and their needs. Just the knowledge that there are preferences should

Figure 3.4 How Do You Like to Learn?

1. Do you like music on while you study, or do you prefer a quiet place?
   Quiet   Music

2. Where would you prefer to work on an assignment?
   Classroom   Desk (home)
   On the floor   At a table
   On a computer

3. If you are not able to complete something, is it because
   You forgot?   You are bored?
   You got distracted?   You need help?

4. Where do you like to sit in class?
   Near the door   Front
   By the wall   Near a window
   Back

5. How do you like to work?
   _____ by yourself
   _____ with a partner
   _____ in a small group

6. Are you more alert in the afternoon? In the evening? In the morning?

7. What classes do you enjoy most and why?
   _____
   _____
   _____

8. Describe how you study. Where? When? How?
   _____
   _____
   _____

9. If you have an assignment due in 2 weeks, how do you plan to complete it?
   _____
   _____
   _____

10. If something is new for you, do you
    Like to have it explained?   Like to read about it?
    Like to watch a video/demonstration?   Like to just try it?

influence teachers' plans for presenting a variety of material and designing practice in the classroom with options and choices.

THINKING PREFERENCES

Anthony Gregorc (1982), at the University of Connecticut, has developed a theory of thinking styles based on two variables: the way we view the world (whether we see the world in an abstract or concrete way) and the way we order the world (in a sequential or random order). Using these variables, Gregorc combines them to create four styles of thinking:

- **Concrete Random Thinkers**, who enjoy experimentation, are also known as *divergent thinkers*. They are eager to take intuitive leaps in order to create. They have a need to find alternate ways of doing things. Thus in the classroom, these thinkers need to be allowed to have opportunities to make choices about their learning and about how they demonstrate understandings. These learners enjoy creating new models and practical things that result from their new learning and concept development.
- **Concrete Sequential Thinkers** are based in the physical world identified through their senses. They are detail oriented, notice details, and recall them with ease. They require structure, frameworks, timelines, and organization to their learning. They like lecture and teacher-directed activities.
- **Abstract Sequential Thinkers** delight in the world of theory and abstract thought. Their thinking processes are rational, logical, and intellectual. They are happiest when involved with their own work and investigation. These learners need to have the time to examine fully the new ideas, concepts, and theories with which they have been presented. They like to support the new information by investigating and analyzing so that the learning makes sense and has real meaning for them.
- **Abstract Random Thinkers** organize information through sharing and discussing. They live in a world of feelings and emotion and learn best when they can personalize information. These learners like to discuss and interact with others as they learn. Cooperative group learning, centers or stations, and partner work facilitate their understanding.

Dr. Robert Sternberg (1996), in his book *Successful Intelligence*, suggests that intelligent people who will be successful in life are able to take information or knowledge and use it in practical, analytical, and creative ways (see Figure 3.5). Learners with different preferences bring to the group their natural abilities to be practical, analytical, and creative. This theory gives all teachers the opportunity to engage and motivate learners to complete a task by offering choice in how they approach a new topic and how they take their learning in different directions. It may also be appropriate to have a variety of learners with different approaches working together. Different ways of thinking are not a detriment to group interaction, but rather a gift when different perspectives are represented and shared. The Common Core State Standards recommend that students use analytical and creative skills to become more capable citizens of the world.

David Kolb (1984) also developed a learning-style profile based on experiential learning, which includes the following four groups:

Figure 3.5   Sternberg's Triarchic Model

Intelligence	What It Means
Practical	These learners stress the usefulness or how knowledge and skills are used in the real world. They appreciate authentic applications.
Analytical	These learners stress looking at the relationship of parts to whole and thorough examination, such as many schools tasks do.
Creative	These learners stress the opportunity to create visions and possibilities related to the concepts and skills.

- **Accommodators.** These students like to try out new things and "shake up" their own and others' "boxes." They like to be creative, they are flexible risk takers, and they want to do things their way.
- **Convergers.** These learners value and want to know only what is useful and relevant to the immediate situation or question. They are good at pulling out and organizing essential information. They like clear goals and specific timelines.
- **Assimilators.** These learners want to investigate, read, research, and learn as much as possible about a topic. They have the patience and tenacity to delve deeply into information, and they enjoy abstract content. They believe that they learn from past experiences and from experts.
- **Divergers.** These students value positive, caring environments with comfortable surroundings. They like to learn from others through conversation and dialogue. They want to explore and seek alternatives, and they are altruistic in their pursuit of learning.

Bernice McCarthy's 4MAT model (McCarthy, 1990; McCarthy & McCarthy, 2006) identifies four learning styles and the type of teaching strategies best suited to each of them: (1) the imaginative learner, (2) the analytical learner, (3) the commonsense learner, and (4) the dynamic learner. Learners are capable of working in all four areas some of the time, but most of us tend to favor one style over all others. The trick for teachers is to provide experiences in the four areas to accommodate all learners and to increase their range of learning styles. It can be useful to view the model as a circle divided into four quadrants that can be used to guide lesson planning and teaching (see Figure 3.6).

- **Type 1: The Imaginative Learner (Experiencing).** These learners seek meaning. They are innovative and imaginative, preferring to learn through feeling and reflecting. Their teachers need to create a reason and provide a rationale for the learning that connects to their own lives and has relevance. Positive relationships and nurturing teachers are important aspects that need to be present in classrooms.
- **Type 2: The Analytical Learner (Conceptualizing).** These learners seek facts. They prefer to learn by watching and thinking. They create concepts and models. They appreciate information and teacher lectures.
- **Type 3: The Commonsense Learner (Applying).** These learners seek usability and practical application and prefer to learn through thinking and trying out. Experimentation and problem solving are processes that intrigue these learners.

Figure 3.6   Suggestions in Bernice McCarthy's 4Mat Model

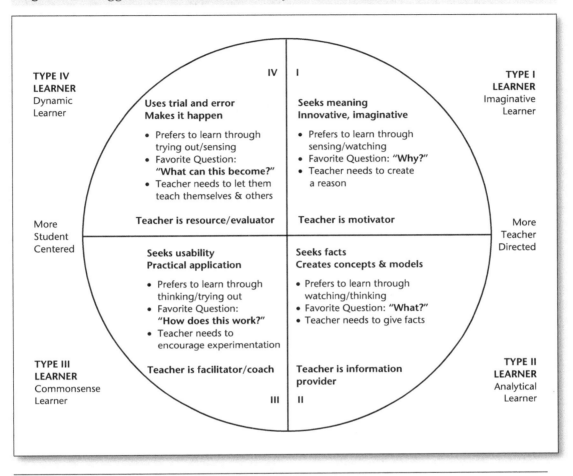

Source: Adapted from McCarthy (1990), McCarthy & McCarthy (2006).

- **Type 4: The Dynamic Learner (Creating).** These learners seek to learn through trial and error and prefer to learn by trying out and sensing. They want to teach themselves and others and to use the teacher as a resource. They are risk takers and prefer self-discovery, disliking rigid routines and methodical tasks.

Silver, Strong, and Perini (2000) and Silver and Perini (2010) outline a model of four learning styles derived from the theories of Carl Jung and Isabel Briggs Myers:

- **Self-Expressive Learners** prefer opportunities for original, flexible, and elaborative thinking. They appreciate teachers who give them choices and facilitate their learning. They are innovative, creative learners.
- **Mastery Learners** prefer opportunities to observe, describe, memorize, and practice new learning to reach mastery. They appreciate teachers who present information and arrange for practice. They enjoy developing mastery of basic skills.
- **Understanding Learners** prefer opportunities to summarize, classify, compare, contrast, and look for cause and effect. They appreciate teachers who provide information and then probe for explanations and reasons behind the facts. They think logically and analytically, seeking evidence to support their learning.

- **Interpersonal Learners** prefer opportunities to socialize, describe feelings, empathize, and provide support and approval. They appreciate teachers who relate the content to them personally so that they can recognize relevance and add meaning to their work.

USING LEARNING AND THINKING PREFERENCES IN THE CLASSROOM

The connections and similarities between and among these various learning styles can be compared using a matrix (see Figure 3.7). Vertically, each column outlines a different research interpretation. Horizontally, each row shows how the different perspectives align with each other.

Figure 3.7 A Matrix of Learning Styles Illustrates Their Connections and Similarities

	Gregorc	Kolb	Silver/Strong/Hanson	4MAT/McCarthy
Beach Ball	**Concrete Random** Divergent Experiential Inventive	**Accommodator** Likes to try new ideas. Values creativity, flexibility, and risk takers.	**Self-Expressive** Feelings to construct new ideas. Produces original and unique materials.	**Type 4 Dynamic** Create and act. Usefulness and application of learning.
Clipboard	**Concrete Sequential** Task oriented Efficient Detailed	**Converger** Values what is useful and relevant, immediacy, and organizing essential information.	**Mastery** Absorbs information concretely, and processes step by step.	**Type 3 Commonsense** Think and do. Active, practical. Make things work.
Microscope	**Abstract Sequential** Intellectual Analytical Theoretical	**Assimilator** Avid readers who seek to learn. Patience for research. Values concepts.	**Understanding** Prefers to explore ideas and use reason and logic based on evidence.	**Type 2 Analytical** Reflect and think. Observers who appreciate lecture methods.
Puppy	**Abstract Random** Imaginative Emotional Holistic	**Diverger** Values positive, caring environments that are attractive, comfortable, and people oriented.	**Interpersonal** Appreciates concrete ideas and social interaction to process and use knowledge.	**Type 1 Imaginative** Feel and reflect. Create and reflect on an experience.

Harvey Silver and colleagues often use metaphorical thinking in their workshops. The analogous use of four items with which most people are familiar (a beach ball, clipboard, microscope, and puppy) can help learners understand the attributes of each style and remember that style by recalling those attributes that relate to the familiar items. Making students aware of these styles, perhaps by asking them about the attributes of beach balls, clipboards, microscopes, and puppies, and having them brainstorm those characteristics will help students understand the differences between styles in the classroom.

After the brainstorming, students can link the profiles to what would be important to provide for these types of learners in the classroom in order for them to be successful in school. For example, beach balls would want to keep moving, be creative, and be free to go where they wish. Therefore if they were in a classroom at school, they would like choice and options in their learning and to have the opportunity to be creative and move freely, using centers and so forth. Students can rank these four items or symbols from 1 to 4, depending on their understanding of themselves. Teachers can point out that we all have some characteristics of each type but that students' top two choices show the way they would prefer to learn and the types of activities that would be most comfortable for them.

Teachers may want to take time to examine what each of the four types could appreciate in the classroom. One group of teachers generated the following list, containing things that they thought the four types would value:

 ### Beach Ball

- Variety of resources
- Adaptive environment
- Various manipulatives
- Choice of activities
- Spontaneity
- Extensions to activities
- Personal freedom

 ### Microscope

- Investigative learning
- Critical thinking
- Verifying information
- Analyzing concepts
- Deep exploration
- Discussions
- Focus on details
- Ownership

 ### Clipboard

- Organization
- Structure
- Visual directions
- Clear closure
- Sequential learning
- Clear procedures
- Consistent routines
- Clear expectations

 ### Puppy

- Comfortable environment
- Encouraging atmosphere
- Supportive grouping
- Safe climate
- Respectful colleagues
- Empathic listeners
- Sensitive peers

It is not as important which style delineator a teacher uses as it is that the teacher recognize the fact that different students have different preferences. The teacher must design the learning so that the diverse populations in the classroom all have their needs satisfied at some point.

MULTIPLE INTELLIGENCES

Howard Gardner's (2004, 2006) theory of multiple intelligences provides us with another frame through which we can observe students and understand how they learn and process information:

> I believe that human cognitive competence is better described in terms of a set of abilities, talents, or mental skills, which I call intelligences. All normal individuals possess each of these skills to some extent; individuals differ in the degree of skill and the nature of their combination. I believe this theory of intelligence may be more humane and more veridical than alternative views of intelligence and that it more adequately reflects the data of human "intelligent" behavior. (Gardner, 2006, p. 6)

Gardner offers us eight alternative intelligences:

1. **Verbal/Linguistic:** reading, writing, speaking, and listening
2. **Logical/Mathematical:** working with numbers and abstract patterns
3. **Visual/Spatial:** working with graphic images, mind mapping, graphic organizers, visualizing, drawing, and exploring the world of color and art
4. **Musical/Rhythmic:** using rhythm, melody, patterned sound, song, rap, dance
5. **Bodily/Kinesthetic:** processing information through touch, movement, dramatics, manipulatives, and using a variety of fine and gross motor skills in everyday life
6. **Interpersonal:** sharing, cooperating, interviewing, relating, and brainstorming with others
7. **Intrapersonal:** working alone, self-paced instruction, individualized projects, and metacognitive thinking
8. **Naturalist:** spending time outdoors, sorting, classifying, and noticing patterns in the world

Finding Gold

One teacher shared with us that she felt she was constantly observing her students trying to identify their strengths in multiple intelligences. She likened it to mining for gold. Teachers in classrooms have been not only recognizing the various intelligences that students possess but also consciously providing learning experiences that include more than the most frequently used verbal and logical intelligences. They consider the notion that when we want to catch fish, we bait the hook with what the fish like, not what the fisherman likes. So in classrooms, teachers should use a variety of teaching and learning strategies as "bait" that will appeal to the learners, not just to the teacher.

"Kidwatching"

Getting to know students is one way of gathering data to build learning profiles for each student. Teachers and students need to know their strengths, in order to enhance self-confidence, as well as areas that need improvement, so goal setting and metacognition can be implemented. Teachers and students may use checklists and questionnaires (see Figures 3.8 through 3.14) to gain insight into students' preferred areas of multiple intelligences.

How Are You Intelligent?

"How Are You Intelligent?" (see Figure 3.8) is a checklist that students and teachers may use to increase personal awareness and understanding of areas of strength, which will increase self-awareness and confidence, and to identify areas that they may need to target for growth. Students may check off the items that are most like themselves and then transfer that information to a bar graph, filling in one cube in each row for each item checked in each intelligence category. The bar graph can then be cut to create each student's "Unique Multiple Intelligences Profile" (see Figure 3.9), which may be used to compare and contrast their profiles with other students with whom they may be working (Fogarty & Stoehr, 1995). This helps students recognize that together they have at least three or four areas of strength and therefore more tools for creativity and problem solving. This activity reinforces the notion that our diversity is our strength. As students learn through experience and reflection on those experiences, their profiles will be forever changing (see also Chapman, 1993).

Student Observations

Observing students as they work and interact helps us know them better. Some classroom teachers set up areas where students choose games or activities for leisure time at noon hour or recess. The types of games they choose gives teachers information about their preferences. For example, some students choose games or activities that involve words and letters, others problems and logic, others creative options, and still others social interaction. Teachers often use clipboards and self-sticking notes to capture observations about students that can be transferred into student profiles (see Figure 3.10) whenever possible.

Logs and Journals

Teachers gain valuable information in logs and journals in which students reflect on their learning and their enjoyment or preference of one learning activity over another. Having students use exit passes as they leave the class can give the teacher immediate feedback on specific topics. Just asking students what they enjoyed, or learned best from, or didn't appreciate gives information that can be valuable in future planning. Teachers can also check for clarification and understanding of material that was examined in class that day by asking what was clear, what was unclear,

Figure 3.8   How Are You Intelligent?

VERBAL/LINGUISTIC INTELLIGENCE	INTRAPERSONAL INTELLIGENCE
• I like to tell jokes, stories, or tales. • Books are important to me. • I like to read. • I often listen to radio, TV, tapes, or CDs. • I write easily and enjoy it. • I quote things I've read. • I like crosswords and word games.	• I know about my feelings, strengths, and weaknesses. • I like to learn more about myself. • I enjoy hobbies by myself. • I enjoy being alone sometimes. • I have confidence in myself. • I like to work alone. • I think about things and plan what to do next.
LOGICAL/MATHEMATICAL INTELLIGENCE	VISUAL/SPATIAL INTELLIGENCE
• I solve math problems easily. • I enjoy math and using computers. • I like strategy games. • I wonder how things work. • I like using logic to solve problems. • I reason things out. • I like to use data in my work to measure, calculate, and analyze.	• I shut my eyes and see clear pictures. • I think in pictures. • I like color and interesting designs. • I can find my way around unfamiliar areas. • I draw and doodle. • I like books with pictures, maps, and charts. • I like videos, movies, and photographs.
INTERPERSONAL INTELLIGENCE	BODILY/KINESTHETIC INTELLIGENCE
• People ask me for advice. • I prefer team sports. • I have many close friends. • I like working in groups. • I'm comfortable in a crowd. • I have empathy for others. • I can figure out what people are feeling.	• I get uncomfortable when I sit too long. • I like to touch or be touched when talking. • I use my hand when speaking. • I like working with my hands on crafts/hobbies. • I touch things to learn more about them. • I think of myself as well coordinated. • I learn by doing rather than watching.
MUSICAL/RHYTHMIC INTELLIGENCE	NATURALIST
• I like to listen to musical selections. • I am sensitive to music and sounds. • I can remember tunes. • I listen to music when studying. • I enjoy singing. • I keep time to music. • I have a good sense of rhythm.	• I enjoy spending time in nature. • I like to classify things into categories. • I can hear animal and bird sounds clearly. • I see details when I look at plants, flowers, and trees. • I am happiest outdoors. • I like tending to plants and animals. • I know the names of trees, plants, birds, and animals.

Figure 3.9   What Is Your Unique Multiple Intelligences Profile?

Word Smart							
Math Smart							
People Smart							
Music Smart							
Self Smart							
Picture Smart							
Body Smart							
Nature Smart							

Source: Adapted with permission from *Integrating Curricula With Multiple Intelligences: Teams, Themes, and Threads,* by Robin Fogarty and Judy Stoehr. © 1995 Corwin. www.corwin.com.

Figure 3.10 Student Profile Based on Teacher Observations

Student Profile	
Observing over time . . .	**Name:**
Verbal/Linguistic	**Intrapersonal**
Logical/Mathematical	**Visual/Spatial**
Interpersonal	**Bodily/Kinesthetic**
Musical/Rhythmic	**Naturalist**

or what questions still need clarification. Figure 3.11 offers a self-reflection tool that students can use in journals as a whole or as individual items over several days. These metacognitive strategies are essential to foster a growth mindset and help students take ownership of their own learning.

In early elementary classrooms, students can use symbols or a "Yes—Maybe—No" checklist (see Figure 3.12) instead of words to indicate their preferences. The teacher may pose questions like those listed on the bottom half of the checklist, and after thinking about each question, the students can draw a face on the appropriate line that shows how they feel about the activity.

As teachers become more aware of students' unique learning preferences and intelligences, they become more able to design learning experiences that appeal to their students' different needs and interests. Because teachers are also unique individuals who tend to have styles of teaching that fit their personal profiles, it is often a stretch to include instructional and assessment tools and strategies that are not in their personal comfort zones.

Teachers need to build repertoires that will engage more learners and honor the diversity in each classroom. The multiple intelligences offer many options for including all eight, where appropriate, in lessons (see Figure 3.13). When teachers use a variety of multiple intelligences processes, they offer diverse learners more opportunities to learn and to show what they know in many ways. Refer to the palette of suggestions to guide lesson planning (see Figure 3.14).

Teachers continually gather data and observe students as the students become more familiar with their unique ways of learning. Teachers then can consciously include a variety of learning and assessment experiences that would appeal and engage a greater number of students. Students will then feel challenged in areas they feel confident pursuing. We realize that with individual learning styles and multiple intelligences profiles, one size of learning could not possibly fit everyone in the classroom. Knowing the learners and consciously and strategically planning to address their styles, intelligences, and learning preferences will increase the chances of engaging them and offering a variety of ways to learn.

Figure 3.11 Eight Intelligences: Self-Reflection Tool Used by Students Individually or With Peers

Complete this page and compare your answers with your partner.

If I could do anything I like, I'd . . . .

Usually, when I have free time I . . . .

My hobbies are . . . .

At school I like to . . . .

The type of things that we do in class I really like are . . . .

I am uncomfortable when people ask me to . . . .

Do you like to work alone or with a group? Why?

Figure 3.12   Yes—Maybe—No Line

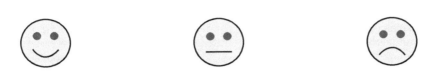

1.

2.

3.

4.

5.

6.

7.

8.

9.

10.

Ask students about a variety of activities that they might have the opportunity to do.

How do you feel about . . .

1.   Drawing and artwork?

2.   Musical activities?

3.   Working with others?

4.   Working alone?

5.   Using numbers?

6.   Writing? Talking?

7.   Dancing, sports, moving while learning?

8.   Solving problems?

9.   Reading?

10.   Thinking about things?

11.   Working with technology?

12.   Being a leader?

Figure 3.13 Focusing on Multiple Intelligences in the Classroom

Definitions	Cultivation of Intelligence	Applications in Classroom
Verbal/Linguistic Uses language to read, write, and speak to communicate	• Play word games for vocabulary • Practice explaining ideas • Tell jokes and riddles • Play trivia games • Make up limericks	Write Report Explain Describe and discuss Interview Label Give and follow directions
Musical/Rhythmic Communicates in rhyme and rhythm	• Interview people about their favorite music • Make up a song about your favorite things • Play "name that tune" • Create a class song • Share poems that are special to you	Chant Sing Raps and songs Beat a rhythm Poetry Limericks
Logical/ Mathematical Uses logic and reason to solve problem	• Introduce graphic organizers to students and let them reflect on their use • Offer logic problems or situations and have students share problem-solving strategies	Advance organizers Graphic organizers Puzzles Debates Critical thinking Graphs and charts Data and statistics
Visual/Spatial Ability to visualize in the mind's eye	• Offer students opportunities to close their eyes and visualize: scenes, processes, and events • Allow and encourage students to add drawings and representations in their work or demonstrate understanding	Draw Create Visualize Paint Imagine Models Describe in detail
Bodily/Kinesthetic Ability to learn and express oneself through the whole body	• Let students role-play processes and events • Create a dance or mime to illustrate new learning • Create gestures or actions that demonstrate new learning	Perform Create Construct Develop Manipulate Dance or mime
Naturalist Ability to recognize and classify	• Provide students with opportunities to classify and examine learning for similar or different attributes • Allow students time for examination and a closer look	Classify, sort Organize using criteria Investigate Analysis Identify, categorize
Intrapersonal Ability to be self-reflective	• Ask students to think about a plan for their assignment or to reflect on the process and set goals for improvement • Introduce journals or reflection time so students reflect on their work and their thinking	Metacognition Logs and journals Independent study Goal setting Positive affirmations Autobiography Personal questions
Interpersonal Ability to work with others	• Practice positive skills of active listening, encouragement • Show appreciation for the "smarts" of others	Group work Partner activities Reciprocal teaching Peer reading, editing, counseling Role-playing Class meetings Conferencing and sharing

Figure 3.14   Suggestions for Using the Eight Multiple Intelligences

Verbal/Linguistic Brainstorm. Organize thoughts. Summarize. Change the beginning or the end. Describe it. Write a blog about it Write an advertisement. Write an editorial. Write a news flash. Prepare a speech. Create copy for a webpage. Develop a campaign platform. Develop a challenging question. Find evidence to support a claim. Use figurative language. Research the inventor or an author. Write a conclusion, summary. Write main idea and supporting details. Develop a book. Record reading or writing. Skim and scan. Write the attributes. Write adjectives or phrases to describe.	**Musical/Rhythmic** Compose a song. Think of a theme song and say why. Write a poem. Create a jingle or slogan. Select sounds to fit. Recognize pitch, tone, timbre. Use background music. Create a beat. Make rhythmic movements. Identify sounds. Identify musical pieces. Interpret a song. Record music. Develop an instrument. Find the background music. Use Songify app to create a song.
Logical/Mathematical Sequence. Design a game. Develop a TV show. Create a timeline. Tell your process. Categorize. Find the missing piece or link. Classify. Rank ideas. Use a matrix. Design a graph. Try a new idea. Survey. Conduct an inventory. Do an Internet search for key words. Research and gather data. Interpret data. Technology world. Gadget use. Compute or calculate.	**Visual/Spatial** Draw a picture or graphic. Make a flip book. Create a photo essay. Create a website. Post a YouTube video. Design a poster. Design a puppet. Make a collage. Illustrate it. Plot on a graphic organizer. Design or create. Associate using color. Use different art media. Interpret a piece of art. Design a book. Sculpt it! Draw a map. Design a diorama. Highlight or tabbing. Develop a character sketch.
Bodily/Kinesthetic Movement. Name its function. Brainstorm. Use your body to interpret meaning. Play a game or sport. Use manipulative. Construct or build.	**Interpersonal** Work with others. Empathetic with others. Work on a group project. Conduct an interview. Discuss with others. Be involved in a conversation. Come to a consensus.

(Continued)

(Continued)

Role-play and post.
Perform.
Act it out.
Mime.
Puppet show.
Show how you know.
Dramatize.
Create simulations.
Interpretive dance.
Do an experiment.
Invent or discover through
   trial and error.
	Give or receive feedback.
	Jigsaw information.
	Be a team member.
	Use a social network to most information about the
	   topic.

Intrapersonal Select personal choice. Work alone. Use metacognitive thinking. Plan a way. Get a strategy. Draw a conclusion of how it makes you feel. Identify likes and dislikes. Make choices. Self-assess. Set goals. Carry through a task. How does it feel? Identify your personal preference. Automaticity. Develop an ejournal. Gather items for a portfolio.	**Naturalist** Surviving. Understand nature. Use nature to work for you. Study science. Explore on the Internet. Apply information to life. Make a personal link and connection from your world. Learn survival needs. Identify scientific method and classifications. Study of land, sea, and air. Make discoveries. Invent. Explore the world.

GENDER DIFFERENCES

Gender differences are another compelling reason to differentiate. There are more than 100 structural differences between the female and male brains. Both genetics and how we are socialized contribute to these differences. Figure 3.15 highlights some of these differences.

So in Classrooms . . .

We should consider these biological differences and respond appropriately. The following suggestions may be taken into account to satisfy and engage males and females in the classrooms.

Provide opportunities for gender-alike groups.

Recognize that girls pay attention and can listen longer than boys, so vary the time.

Provide movement with smooth and limited transitions.

Recognize that girls have a nurturing, bonding nature, and respect that. Also, they are often teacher pleasers.

Connect more at a verbal, emotional level for girls.

Provide healthy, collaborative competition.

Offer choice of tasks to satisfy the spatial and verbal learners.

Provide both colorful materials and multimedia to satisfy all learners.

Figure 3.15   Gender Differences

Areas of Differences	Female Brains	Male Brains
Frontal lobe	There is a lot of activity in the frontal cortex, and it develops earlier than a boy's frontal lobe. Thus girls can attend and focus longer.	Boys may be labeled as learning disabled with behavioral disorders because the frontal lobe is less developed and they are more impulsive.
Visual/spatial	Girls' brains have more cortical emphasis on emotions and verbal processing. Girls use many more words than boys.	Boys' brains have more areas dedicated to spatial functioning.
P cells and M cells	Type P ganglion cells in the visual system are more prevalent, and girls are drawn more to color and fine sensory activity.	Type M ganglion cells in the optical and neural area are greater in boys. Boys rely on pictures and movement when they write.
Neural rest states	Girls' brains stay active even when they are bored. They can still make notes, listen, and write.	Boys' brains take more rest breaks throughout the day and need physical stimuli to stay focused and engaged.
Natural aggression	Girls are less competitive and aggressive than boys because of more oxytocin. Girls desire to bond and please others.	Boys are more aggressive and competitive naturally for several neural and chemical reasons. Boys have less oxytocin and are more impulsive and less interested in the bonding malleability.
Cross-brain functions	Girls have larger corpus callosums, there is more cross-talk between left and right hemispheres, and they are better at multitasking.	Boys compartmentalize more and prefer to be more linear in tasks. They take more time to transition between tasks.

Source: Adapted from Gurian & Stevens (2005).

CULTURAL DIFFERENCES

Gay (2000) defines culturally responsive teaching as using the cultural knowledge, prior experiences, and performance styles of diverse students to make learning more appropriate and effective for them; it teaches to and through the strengths of these students. It is obvious as we look at classrooms that there are fewer and fewer White students who may not know how to navigate school. It is important to recognize that all students—regardless of race or ethnicity—bring their culturally influenced cognition, behavior, and dispositions with them to school. It is important that we acknowledge their culture and make an effort to understand the beliefs, values, attitudes, norms, and predispositions to help them feel valued, confident, and included in the classroom. Students can't learn in an environment that does not match their schema and/or connect with how they view the world.

Western culture, with its particular values and beliefs, may clash with others.

Social as well as cognitive behaviors may differ.

Silence versus talking may be the norm.

Individual versus collaborative activities may be valued.

Although we may know about general impressions of a culture, the student may not fit the mold exactly. There are generalities but also particulars. Interacting, observing, discussing, and questioning students will help teachers better understand the individuals' needs.

As teachers respect the students' cultures and tries to include materials, provide resources, and build connections and bridges between different cultures, students become more connected to the learning and parents feel more at ease interacting with the school. Differentiating the content and materials may better meet the needs of students of other cultures.

POP CULTURE DIFFERENCES

Not only is ethnicity important but also connecting and relating to what students attend to in their personal world of pop culture. Finding out this information may help connect, respect, and engage learners by bridging the learning to their world.

Whether it is teen idols, singers, characters, video games, or trends, students love to know that teachers know and care about their world outside the school. By having the teacher respect and connect the learning to these real-world interests, students will feel recognized and be more responsive to school.

If a teacher is not connecting with a student, the teacher may want to build a full student profile to carefully examine how he or she might plan more thoughtfully to motivate and engage. Building a full profile for each student may be overwhelming, so start small. Students may help build their own profiles and reflect daily or several times a week using journals and exit passes to suggest what they enjoyed, found lacking (boring), or would rather have done.

Beginning to observe and collect data about the student and consciously responding to that by adjusting lessons and providing choice will help you know your students' preferences and interests.

Chapter 3
Reflections

In your professional learning communities you may want to discuss and investigate some of the following.

1. How do you get to know your students? What methods do you use?

2. How do you stimulate your students' strongest intelligences? How do you encourage students to cultivate their other intelligences?

3. How could you develop awareness about multiple intelligences with students and parents?

4. Use the suggestions in Figure 3.14 to check that learning styles and multiple intelligences are varied.

5. As you examine your lessons and units, are the needs of male and female students respected?

6. What cultures are represented, and what do you know about them?

7. Does your curriculum include opportunities to connect with all cultures present in your classroom and school?

8. What are the pop culture interests of your students? What bridges can you build?

4

Assessing the Learner

JUST AS ONE SIZE OF LEARNING DOESN'T FIT ALL, ONE SIZE OF assessment doesn't suit, either. These diverse learners we serve all have had prior experiences and come with different understandings related to content and skills (Donovan & Bransford, 2005).

We can hold up clothing to see how it might look, but until we put it on, we don't know what changes need to be made. We may need a new size or a different style or color. So in assessing the learning, we need different approaches to check the fit and adjust the learning.

We in education tend to banter about the terms *assessment*, *evaluation*, and *grading* without necessarily having clearly distinctive definitions for each term. *Assessment* is often referred to as the gathering of data, *evaluation* is the judging of merits, and *grading* is assigning values to letters or numbers for reporting purposes (Rolheiser, Bower, & Stevahn, 2000).

Assessment terms have broadened over the last decade. Following is a glossary of terms.

GLOSSARY OF TERMS

Authentic Assessment: a form of assessment whereby students perform a real-world task to show depth of understanding of concepts and application of skills.

E-portfolios: a digital collection of a student's work gathered over an assigned period of time to reveal strengths, areas of need, progress, and outcomes.

Formative Assessment: the ongoing process of gathering and interpreting data to plan instruction and to gauge growth.

Portfolio: a showcase of evidence of an individual's work samples.

Pre-assessment: a formative assessment given at the beginning of a topic or unit of study to establish prior knowledge, readiness, interests, and preferences.

Summative Assessment: the final evaluation (value of or sum) that shows the student's mastery level and understanding of the learning at the end of the instructional period.

FORMATIVE ASSESSMENT

Formative assessment is assessment **for** learning (Stiggins, Arter, Chappuis, & Chappuis, 2006). It includes both pre-assessment and ongoing assessment to judge what students know at a given point in time and what needs to be done next to help students achieve the standard.

Differentiation is driven by data. You can't make instructional decisions without considering what students know, can do, are interested in, and prefer. Assessment drives instruction: pre-assessment first and then ongoing formative assessment throughout the learning.

With clear objectives targeted, ongoing assessment is necessary to keep tailoring the instruction and marking the progress based on the data (Earl, 2003).

Summative assessment is used at the end of the learning period to check the "sum" of the learning that has taken place. Comparing the pre-assessment and summative assessment shows the growth of the student.

One of the first things that needs to be done is pre-assessment, to find out what students already know or can do (prior knowledge). It takes time to do quality pre-assessments, but it can be a very worthwhile process. Planning for individual and group needs is easier when the teacher investigates and discovers what a student knows, how the student feels about the topic, and what he or she is interested in learning during the unit of study.

PURPOSES OF PRE-ASSESSMENT

Assessing student knowledge prior to the learning experience helps the teacher find out a variety of things:

- What the student already knows (prior knowledge) about the unit being planned
- What standards, objectives, concepts, and skills the student understands
- What further instruction and opportunities for mastery are needed
- What requires reteaching or enhancement
- What areas of interests and feelings are in the different areas of the study
- How to set up flexible groups: T (total), A (alone), P (partner), S (small)

When teaching with high achievement as a goal, one important aspect of assessing learners is finding out what the students already know. This knowledge is based on their prior learning and experiences. By doing a pre-assessment, teachers can plan curriculum and design instruction to meet the needs of the total class as well as individuals. Written tests are one form of pre-assessment.

Try this handy tip! Administer the pretest 2 or 3 weeks before the information is to be taught. The test needs to vary in types of questions for an accurate assessment. That gives the teacher time to plan for the novice to the expert and those along the way. By administering the test early, the seeds of excitement have been planted about all the interesting things the students will be learning. Students need to realize that it is through experiences that they learn. They may be at a novice level of knowing because of lack of experience and opportunity. This is sometimes difficult for a student to admit. One must realize that the pre-assessment tools provide information for planning what the individual needs and that no one is expected to be at the expert level in everything being taught.

When learners know the information, they may be allowed to move on to another dimension of the unit of study. For those who have not had exposure to the information prior to the pre-assessment, this allows the teacher to provide an experience for them.

One way to get this point across to students is to name some sports, hobbies, or free-time favorites and find those who are experienced and those who do not know much about them. These students have other areas of interests and expertise. We are all smart, just in different ways. For instance, a star football player knows all the plays of the game and practices for hours. Some of us who attend the football games know the basic rules, and then there are others who do not know anything about the game of football. This has nothing to do with their intelligence; it has to do with their experience, their talents, their interests, and being in the right place at the right time.

Some children in first grade may have difficulty with the concepts related to adding and subtracting numbers. Yet when you get to the money unit, you find that they have been going to the store, spending money, and getting change. These children are in fact able to use the principles of adding and subtracting. Experience and survival have taught them this. Other students may not have had these same experiences.

Pretest

- Include questions or tasks to assess all the outcomes in the entire unit of study.
- Include simple-to-complex and concrete-to-abstract understandings.
- Arrange test questions in groupings that relate to the same standards so that the data, when examined, will clearly indicate knowledge or gaps in knowledge.
- Recall facts.
- Ask students to use the information to show another way, form, or situation.
- Interpret information such as charts and graphs.
- Allow drawing, interpreting, or demonstrating.
- Ask open-ended questions to elicit more information.

Informal Pre-assessment

- Demonstrate with manipulatives, if appropriate, to show application.
- Use interest surveys.
- Use dialogue to find out what students want to learn and how they feel about the topic.
- Analyze the pretest data so you can make planning decisions.

Rank Scores

- Determine appropriate uses of flexible grouping.
- Form timelines for the unit of study or topic.
- Discover the number of students at different levels of mastery.
- Then identify and determine what level of mastery students have reached for the standards, concepts, and skills that will be taught:

   __Beyond expectation (understand, apply, can transfer to other situations)
   __Mastered (a basic understanding)
   __Approaching mastery
   __Introductory, novice, or beginning stage

Then a learning plan can be developed for students at each level of mastery.

There are other effective tools and strategies to use to pre-assess students' knowledge. Emotions and feelings play a large role in the way in which a student learns information. When a person has had a bad experience in the past and is learning or doing something that triggers that memory, there is a barrier formed that inhibits the new learning. When the experience is a quality one with a purpose, a positive impact, and a great experience, the learner feels open to learning more and experiencing more with the topic. These pre-assessment tools relate feelings, emotional links, and knowledge gathered from past experiences. This can have a strong impact on the present learning. The following are some examples of more informal pre-assessment tools that can be used at the beginning of lessons to open mental files and find out students' predispositions.

SAMPLES OF INFORMAL PRE-ASSESSMENTS

Squaring Off

This very successful pre-assessment tool involves the total group.

1. In each corner of the room, place a card containing one of the following words or phrases, which are effective ways to group according to learner knowledge (see Figures 4.1 and 4.2):

Rarely ever	Sometimes	Often	I have it!
Dirt road	Paved road	Highway	Yellow Brick Road
I know very little	I know some	I know a lot	I know all about this!

2. Tell the students to go to the corner of the room that matches their place in the learning journey.

3. Participants go to the corner of the room that most closely matches their own learning status and discuss what they know about the topic or event and why they chose to go there.

Figure 4.1 Squaring Off Sample at Sea

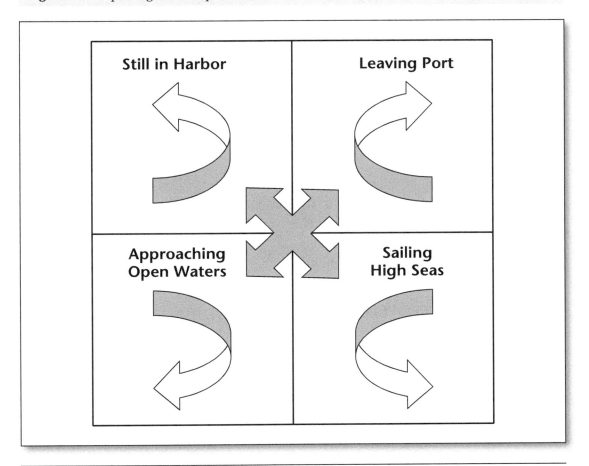

Variations of Squaring Off

Poster paper is provided for the group to write down what they know. Since the first group has little or no background knowledge, they can generate questions or statements about what they want to learn.

Three Corners

Post the following signs in three designated sections of the room.

| Know little or none | Know some | Know this |
| Do not know how | Can explain some | Can explain it |

Follow the same procedure as in Squaring Off.
Note: It is sometimes helpful for students to write down their choice and why they selected that one before going to the designated area.

Boxing

1. Getting to the Heart of the Matter

Draw a box in the center of a piece of paper. Draw a smaller box inside the first box.

- Outside Box:

  What do I know about this topic?

- Inside Box:

  What do I want to learn? or

  What is my goal?

2. Gift of Success

- Outside Box: Write one of the following:

  What else do I know about this topic?

  How does it fit?

  What does this have to do with _____?

- Inside Box:

  Draw a model or picture of the topic.

  Create a graphic organizer to explain the topic.

Figure 4.2 Squaring Off Sample on Land

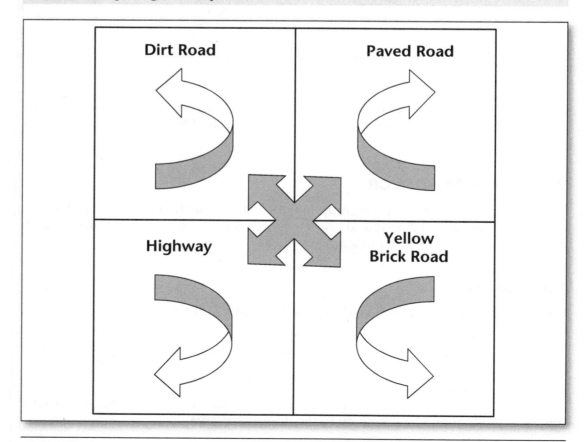

- Middle of the Box:
   Summarize: Write a sentence to explain your thinking.

Variations

- Use different shapes, or give the students a choice of shapes.
- Use as a total-group, small-group, or individual activity.
- Keep adding information throughout the unit to see how much they are learning.
- Do another one as a post-assessment. Place side by side, and reflect on growth.

Responders

Responders are used to allow each student to answer a question. Teachers often use clickers or individual wipe-off boards for this activity. The following is another way to assess what students know about an upcoming topic, skill, or standard. The teacher asks the question, gives the appropriate wait time, and then says, "Cards up!" The teacher receives an instant view of individual reaction as well as an overall view of students who know it and those who do not. Remember, this is an informal assessment.

Yes/No Responder Cards

Yes/No cards may be set up as one-sided or two-sided cards.

Using One-Sided Yes/No Cards

- Give students two blank note cards or pieces of paper. Ask them to write Yes on one and No on the other.
- When a question is asked, the students should hold up a card—Yes if they understand, No if they do not understand.

Examples:

1. Ask the students about vocabulary words for an upcoming unit. Give a word, and ask students to show the Yes card if they know the word and its definition or the No card if they do not know the word and its definition.
2. Ask someone who is showing a Yes card to define the word. This way, the students realize you will be checking their responses.
3. Use some of the most interesting information and words from the upcoming unit to build up anticipation about the topic.
4. Remind students that if they do not know these words, they will be learning more about them in the upcoming unit.
   - Get creative and customize phrases for your class to write on the cards. Some alternative phrases and symbols might be *Got It!* (Yes) and *Not a Clue* (No), or plus (Yes) and minus (No) signs.

Using Two-Sided Yes/No Cards

Teachers may prefer to use two-sided Yes/No cards. In this case, students or teachers can prepare the cards, writing Yes at the top of each card and No underneath it on both sides of the card. When the teacher asks the question, the student holds up the card, pinching the side of the card next to the selected answer. Advantages of two-sided cards include the following:

- When the student holds up the Yes/No card, everyone in the class can view the correct answer on both sides of the card.
- The student can view both Yes and No answers before responding to the teacher's question.
- The teacher can assess the student's finger movements. For example, some students will go right for the answer and pinch, while others move their fingers back and forth, deciding which one is the correct answer. This shows the teacher which students are secure and know the answer and which are still unsure.

Examples of Responder Cards for the Content Areas

Responder cards can also be customized to show subject-specific concepts in the content areas. These can be used before, during, and after the learning for checkpoints and reviews. Each time, the students are showing what they know, and the quick-view analysis can be an excellent formative assessment resource for the students as well as the teacher. The following are some examples of responder cards to use across the content areas.

Math

- add, subtract, multiply, divide
- square, circle, trapezoid, rectangle
- prime, composite

Social Studies

- Asia, Africa, North America
- plebeians, counsel, dictator
- north, south, east, west
- farm, desert, rain forest

Science

- invertebrate, vertebrate
- land, sea, air
- hypothesis, problem, conclusion
- sink, float

Language Arts

- explicit, implicit
- noun, verb, adjective
- nonfiction, fiction
- subject, predicate

Arts and Music

- classical, disco, country
- string, percussion, horn
- renaissance, baroque, modern
- watercolor, oils, chalk

All Subjects

- cause, effect
- fact, opinion
- beginning, middle, end
- understand, do not understand
- yes, no, some
- happy, so-so, sad

Variations

- Give a card to a set of partners or a small group of learners instead of one to each student. The question is given. Then assign consensus discussion time. This is a time when students decide on their answer and why it is right while coming to consensus. Say, "1, 2, 3, show me!" and one of the partners shows the answer.
- Make sure in making the two-sided card that the word on the back is right behind the same word on the front. This way when the student pinches the answer, he or she is looking at the answer and the teacher and peers can also see the student's choice.

Graffiti Fact

Create a Graffiti Board of Facts. Post all the things the class knows about the topic of study:

- What we knew
- What we learned
- What we want to learn next

Give students time to process and think about the answers. Encourage them to write down their answers before sharing with the group. Let students answer the questions alone at first and jot down their answers. In addition, urge students to write their own answers on the Graffiti Board of Facts to foster ownership of the answers.

Variations

- This tool can be used as an ongoing assessment during the learning as well as before the learning.
- Post this 1–3 weeks before teaching the information so the students have time to add what they know but also investigate the topic and add what they are learning before the unit begins.

SURVEYS AT WORK

Construct Quality Surveys

Teachers know the goal, the purpose, and the information that is to be learned. Survey often, because students' interests change as they grow. These tools will teach you so much about the learners in your classroom! See Figures 4.3–4.6.

The surveys may help you find out about the pre-knowledge or experience that students have with an upcoming unit (content surveys). They may help you design

Figure 4.3 Sample Interest Survey Questions

	Rarely Ever	Sometimes	Most of the Time
1. I like to make up songs.	_____	_____	_____
2. I like to try things that are hard to do.	_____	_____	_____
3. Brain puzzles hold my interest.	_____	_____	_____
4. I like to take things apart and reassemble them.	_____	_____	_____
5. I enjoy creating.	_____	_____	_____
6. I need manipulatives to learn.	_____	_____	_____
7. I am a follower.	_____	_____	_____
8. I am a leader.	_____	_____	_____
9. I prefer to work alone.	_____	_____	_____
10. I like to read.	_____	_____	_____
11. I prefer to work with others.	_____	_____	_____
12. I like to draw my own pictures.	_____	_____	_____
13. I can see visual images in my head.	_____	_____	_____
14. I have at least one pet.	_____	_____	_____
15. I enjoy animals.	_____	_____	_____
16. I would rather be outside than inside.	_____	_____	_____
17. I would rather be inside than outside.	_____	_____	_____
18. I like school.	_____	_____	_____
19. I do not like school.	_____	_____	_____
20. School would be better if . . .	_____	_____	_____
21. If I have free time, I prefer to	_____	_____	_____
a. _____	_____	_____	_____
b. _____	_____	_____	_____
c. _____	_____	_____	_____
22. I do not like _____ because _____.	_____	_____	_____
23. Additional Comments	_____	_____	_____
a. _____	_____	_____	_____
b. _____	_____	_____	_____

Figure 4.4 Math Interest Survey

Name: _____

Address: _____

Home Phone: _____

Date: _____

Course: _____

Please help me get to know you better.

1. My top two or three favorite activities are _____

2. Other activities that I like to do are _____

3. My favorite subject is _____

4. In my free time, I _____

5. On TV, I like to watch _____

6. The music I listen to is _____

7. I think a teacher should _____ and _____

8. My favorite movies are _____ and _____

9. I like my family because _____

10. I dislike school because _____

11. I like school because _____

12. Friends are important because _____

13. The most interesting person whom I have met is _____ because
_____

14. My chores at home are _____

15. My job outside of school is _____. How often? _____

16. I volunteer at _____. How often? _____

17. If I had $500, I would _____

18. I am in this math class because _____

19. I think this class will be (easy/difficult) because _____

20. I am excited about this class because _____

21. I am fearful of this class because _____

22. The things I will do in this class to be successful are _____

23. The things that may prevent me from being successful are _____

24. Something that I want you to know about me is _____

25. Any additional comments: _____

Figure 4.5 Foreign Language Interest Inventory (Getting to Know You)

Name: _____

Age: _____

Date: _____

Class: _____

Please help me get to know you better.

1. My top two or three favorite activities are _____

2. Other activities that I like to do are _____

3. My favorite subject is _____

4. In my free time, I _____

5. On TV, I like to watch _____

6. The music I listen to is _____

7. I think a teacher should _____ and _____

8. My favorite movies are _____ and _____

9. I like my family because _____

10. I dislike school because _____

11. I like school because _____

12. Friends are important because _____

13. The most interesting person whom I have met is _____because

    _____

14. My chores at home are _____

15. If I had $500, I would _____

16. I am in this Spanish class because _____

17. I think this class will be (easy/difficult) because _____

18. I am excited about this class because _____

19. I am fearful of this class because _____

20. The things I will do in this class to be successful are _____

21. The things that may prevent me from being successful are _____

22. Something that I want you to know about me is _____

23. Any additional comments: _____

Figure 4.6   Pre-assessment of Content Survey

Directions: Write what you know about each of the topics about the country of _____. We will be studying this soon.

Focus: Study of a Country Such as Canada or Mexico

- History
- Industry
- Beliefs
- Government
- Celebrations, festivals, holidays, and rites
- Geography and location

Students may use a grid to organize their information and use pictures, symbols, and words.

History	Industry	Beliefs
Government	Celebrations	Geography

A Four-Corner Pre-assessment may be used to find out or assess a student's prior knowledge. The following example is only one way to get information. You could put any questions in the grid that would give you the information you want. This may be given out as a ticket a week or two before the unit of study would commence.

Something you know about reptiles.	What are two questions about reptiles?
What would be a good project about reptiles?	With whom would you like to work?

performance tasks related to students' preferences or ratings (preference or interest surveys). They also may give you suggestions for classroom configuration and grouping (social surveys).

Variations

- Get the learners involved! Establish a Survey Question Box for students to generate questions to be asked.
- Insert some of the survey questions or lead-ins at the end of an assignment or test. You continue to learn more about students, and this is a useful time filler when the assignment is completed early.
- Use the responder cards to answer survey questions that fit the format.

FORMATIVE ASSESSMENT TOOLS TO USE DURING THE LEARNING

As students are working, we need to offer opportunities for feedback from teachers, from peers, and through self-reflection. Without feedback, people cannot improve. If we wait until the end of the learning, it may be too late and incorrect information or skills may have been developed. The following strategies are engaging ways to assess student progress informally throughout the learning process.

Thumb It

Have students respond with the position of their thumbs to get an assessment of their understanding.

Where am I now in my understanding of _____?

a. Upside	b. Onside (sideways)	c. Downside
Know a lot	Know some	Know very little

Variations

- Remember, this can be used when students are standing in line. It is quiet and keeps students engaged during times when they are waiting.

- This tool can be used to assess an individual's, partners', or a small group's progress in completing a task. This signals where the group is in the work schedule, who needs help, and who needs something to do during these last few minutes.

Upside	Onside	Downside
Finished	Need just a few more minutes	Half-way there

- Use only two! This signal can be used when students first start to work on an assignment and need clarification of directions, explanation of a term or concept, or material.

Upside	Downside
Ready to work	Need help!

- Instead of thumb movements, use other body movements such as stand, bend, or sit to reveal understanding level. This provides a stretch before beginning the assignment.

Fist of Five

Have students use their hands to show their levels of understanding. Showing all five fingers indicates the highest level of understanding.

How well do I know this?

1 2 3 4 5

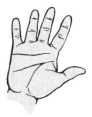

5. I know it so well, I could explain it to anyone.

4. I can do it alone.

3. I need some help.

2. I could use more practice.

1. I am beginning to understand.

Variation

- On a scale of 1 to 3, where are you with understanding:

    1. Completing a task,

    2. Having the resources or materials needed, or

    3. Ready to work.

Face the Fact

1. Have students draw a happy face, a straight face, and a sad face on individual note cards.

2. State a fact related to the topic that can be answered with an emotion.

3. Ask students to hold up the card that matches the emotion.

4. Make motions with your hands to imitate the facial emotions. Curve up for the happy face, flat for the straight face, or curve down for the sad face.

Variation

- Use the happy, straight, and sad face note cards to assess students' understanding of inference. This can be used with characters from fact or fiction.

    a. How did the character feel?
    b. How did the others around the character feel?
    c. How would you feel if you were in that same situation?

Reaching for the Top

1. Tell students to extend one arm straight up in the air.

2. Instruct students to move the opposite hand up that arm as if it were a gauge marked with a 2–4–6–8 scale. Number 2 is at the shoulder, numbers 4 and 6 moving up the arm, and number 8 is at the fingers pointing to the ceiling. This makes learning a cheer celebration!

As each student positions his or her hand against the upraised arm, do a quick scan of the class to check for understanding.

Variation

• Students put their bended arm on the floor or the desk. They use their other hand to mark where they are in their understanding. Start at the elbow, moving out to the finger tips, and assign 2, 4, 6, 8 spots. It is a human Likert scale.

Speedometer Reading

1. Tell students to imagine the speedometer on a car, or draw one on the board. Explain that the speedometer tells how fast the car is moving. The car starts off at 0 miles per hour. Its maximum speed is 100 miles per hour.

2. Have students lay one arm on top of the other with hands touching elbows.

3. Ask students to move the arm that is on top to show a "speed" between 0 and 100. Students show how well they understand or how much they know by indicating the speed on the dial. For example, the student who understands a lot will show 100 miles per hour. The student who knows a little might show 30 miles per hour. Gauge students' understanding by checking the speedometers.

Variation

• Have students find a personal space to respond. This gives feedback plus needed exercise.

Run quickly in place	Walk in place normally	Creep along slowly
I fully understand.	I just about have it.	I am lost!

REFLECTIONS AFTER THE LEARNING

Reflecting on learning is an important step in metacognition. Encourage students to think about what they have learned by using some of these activities.

Wraparounds

1. Participants form a circle.

2. Each individual takes a turn telling . . .

a. Something the student will use from information or activities learned today
b. Something the student will remember from today
c. A significant AHA! from this session
d. I have learned _____
e. I hope to learn _____

Variations

- Form smaller community circles; each person shares a highlight from the day's learning.
- Students write down three important learning discoveries. They join the wraparound and cannot repeat one that has already been said by another circle member. This adds a competitive game edge to the activity, and also more ideas will be generated.

Talking Topic

1. Form A/B partners.

2. A tells a fact to B.

3. B gives another fact back.

4. Partners keep swapping facts back and forth.

Variation A

- Each student writes two important things he or she has learned. Form A/B partners. A shares one thing he or she has learned. B shares one thing he or she has learned. A shares the other important item learned. B shares the other important item learned.

Variation B

- Form A/B partners. A starts discussing a topic, concept, or standard being studied. The teacher gives a signal, such as a hand clap. B takes up the discussion where A left off. The teacher claps again, and A continues the discussion. The process is repeated as many times as necessary. Before the last turn, the teacher claps and says, "Now bring this to closure."

Conversation Circles

1. Form a conversation circle with a group of three students.

2. Ask students to assume A, B, or C names.

3. A starts talking and continues until given the signal to stop.

4. B continues with the topic.

5. C picks up the topic.

6. Continue until there are no more facts or ideas to add to the topic.

Donut

1. Draw a donut shape.

2. On the outside, write, "I am learning."

3. On the inside, write, "I know."

4. Ask students to share what they know about the topic. Write their responses on the donut.

Variation

- Students form inside and outside circles to create a donut shape. The students on the inside circle face the students on the outside. Each student shares what he or she knows. The inside circle moves clockwise, and the outside moves counter clockwise to continue sharing.

Rotation Reflection

1. Post charts around the room with a related topic written on each sheet.

2. Assign small groups to each location. Encourage groups to share ideas and views on the topic written on the chart.

3. Have a recorder fill in the chart with the great ideas generated.

4. Give a signal for the groups to stop talking. Ask the groups to move to the next chart and respond to that topic.

5. Groups continue around the room, visiting each chart in turn and adding ideas.

6. When all groups have visited all the charts, take time to review. At the chart they visit last, ask each small group to consolidate the information and report it to the whole group.

Paper Pass

This activity uses several large pieces of chart paper.

1. Place a different subject heading at the top of each piece of chart paper.

2. Have each group brainstorm and write down what they know about the topic.

3. Each group passes the paper to another group.

4. The second group reads all that has been written, then writes down what else they know about the topic.

5. The second group passes the paper to another group, who also adds to the sheet.

6. The process continues until all groups have contributed to all the subjects.

7. On the last pass, the group finds references for the statements on the chart paper.

8. Instruct students to place a page number and/or source beside each reference.

9. Share and post all the papers.

Draw It!

1. Each set of partners needs a large piece of poster paper and a marker.

2. Partners discuss and come to consensus on an important scene from the study.

3. After deciding, the first student starts the drawing.

4. The second student adds to the picture.

5. The partners swap the marker back and forth until the picture is complete.

6. Show students how to use the picture as a graphic organizer.

7. Instruct the students to brainstorm and write each fact learned about the topic around the picture.

8. Periodically during the study of the unit, have partners add more facts around the drawing.

9. Encourage students to use the drawing as a review before a test or an "open-picture" test.

More Ideas!

Select the items from the following list that are appropriate. Create a Data Board, leaving room for feedback from the students in each section chosen. Students respond to the appropriate question, and their answers are posted. They can keep adding information to the board during the unit.

B   What I Brought

W   What I Want

L   Learnings for Me

S   Suggestions for Next Time

Q   Questions I Have

G   Guesses

P   Pluses

M   Minuses

I   Insights

R   Requests

F   Favorites

D   Dislikes

T   Teach Me!

- Journaling: Students need time allotted to write journal entries about their requests, comments, questions, and reflections
- Plotting data on a variety of graphic organizers
- Polls and interviews
- Conferences
- Performances
- Pre- and posttests
- Portfolios

Grand Finale Comment

Give students a task to do as they are leaving the class. This is the Grand Finale Comment. These comments can give you feedback about student learning, the difficulties groups or individuals encountered, and students' feelings about the situations. Try some of the prompts listed below.

Individual

- Today I learned . . . Tomorrow I need . . .
- Today I felt . . . because . . .
- I would color today [name color] because . . .
- I hope we . . . next.
- One word to describe today is . . .
- I felt like a [name animal] during the . . . because . . .

Group

- Our group was great today when we . . .
- Tomorrow we are going to . . .
- A theme song for our work today would be . . .

ONGOING FORMATIVE AUTHENTIC ASSESSMENT TASKS

An *authentic* and often *complex task* requires that students perform in a realistic, real-world context. It usually engages and motivates student, giving them a purpose for creating rather than reproducing knowledge and understanding over time (Burke, 2009; Prestidge & Williams Glaser, 2000; Wiggins & McTighe, 1998). This may be part of an instructional activity, such as a project, ill-structured problem or dilemma, demonstration, presentation, or role-playing event. The students are asked to demonstrate mastery in ways that simulate a real situation. Therein, the knowledge and skills are practiced and applied, and mastery is shown or demonstrated in a way students can convey it best. Often collaboration and higher order thinking are built in.

In classrooms everywhere, teachers are using authentic strategies to develop the skills addressed in the Common Core State Standards. They also use authentic tools to assess the standards, matching the learning to the assessment. For example, when students work on a project, they are assessed on their work throughout the development of the project as well as on their final report on the project.

Usually a rubric or checklist is developed and used throughout the entire process, so that the student, the parents, and the teacher understand the criteria and expectations and can assess progress along the way.

Portfolios also are now used in many classes, as vehicles for reflection, ongoing conversations, and goal setting between and among students, teachers, and parents.

Formative assessment should provide ongoing feedback as a necessary component of the learning process, not something that happens at the end of the learning. It has been said that feedback is often too little, too late, too vague, presented in the wrong form, and therefore lacking in impact (Jensen, 1998a, p. 54). Feedback must be specific and not just "Good job." "You did a good job using capitals, and now you need to focus on using commas and periods in your sentences" is specific feedback commenting on successful tasks and pointing out next steps or needs. It should provide the same quality a coach would give to improve an athlete's performance. Our challenge is to find ways to facilitate ongoing feedback for students that will increase their chances to continue to grow and improve their learning.

Black and Wiliam (2009) found that, when researching the impact of grades on learning, grades alone did not improve learning and success. Feedback, along with grades, is not very effective either. When students got a grade and feedback on a paper or assignment, they paid more attention to the grade and how they ranked with other students rather than considering the feedback and setting a goal to improve. Students who received only ongoing, specific feedback did up to 60% better than other students who were given grades.

Often benchmark or externally created structured assessments (often mistakenly referred to as formative assessment) to check on student progress are not as helpful, as they do not provide detailed enough information. More precision is needed to give valuable feedback to students or to inform teachers as to appropriate instructional decisions (McMillan, 2007; Popham, 2006; Shepard, 2006).

Assessments for Authentic Performances

Examples of assessment tools include rubrics, anecdotal notes, checklists, journal entries, samples of student work, self-evaluation, and conferences. These tools are used to assess various types of learning activities, from role-playing to projects. Learning needs to be the goal, but making the appropriate grade is often the main focus. Conveying an accurate portrait of students as learners is a complex task.

For example, students are asked to work a problem in math. Then they might be asked to draw the problem and then explain the problem to someone else. In reading, students might be asked to read about a character at a certain point in the text. Then they might be asked to draw the character and put the character in the setting described in the text. Another time, they could be asked to role-play that character or find the background music to depict the character's feelings during a particular part of the story.

These are authentic strategies that allow the learner to interpret meaning. Some of these could be assessed with a written form, but most would need an authentic assessment tool to match the authentic task. Figure 4.7 lists tasks and products that teachers can use to assess student learning in more authentic ways.

Clear expectations and criteria need to be communicated up front so that students know the target and work toward it.

Figure 4.7 Performance Assessment Examples

Verbal/ Linguistic	Visual/ Spatial	Bodily/ Kinesthetic	Musical/ Rhythmic	Logical/ Mathematical
Plan a trip. Conduct a panel. Create a talk show. Teach a lesson. Complete a portfolio. Conduct a survey. Write an editorial.	Make a mural. Create a brochure. Create a costume. Design a PowerPoint. Draw an illustration.	Conduct a demonstration. Develop a role-play. Create a puppet play. Demonstrate an experiment.	Choreograph a dance. Write lyrics to a song. Create a poem. Write a rap. Create a cheer. Create a CD with theme songs.	Create a flow chart. Create a time line. Show step-by-step process. Sequence of events. Write a "how-to" manual.

For a more accurate report, the teacher can include a grade, a portfolio to show the evidence to support the grade, a comment section with specific data about individual performance, and a parent conference for students and teachers to discuss areas of needs and areas of mastery.

Student Choices

Teachers are experimenting with a variety of ways to allow students to show what they know. One teacher has been quite creative in designing tests. She offered students two options. The first option was traditional, consisting of 20 right and wrong answers to volume and area problems, with memorized formulas and no calculator. Points were given for correct formula, answer, and label of answer. The second option allowed calculator use and a formula sheet for students during the test. The problems were applications to real life, thus not perfect math numbers. The shapes were real ice cream cones or lawn sprinklers and showed the actual uses of formulas in our everyday lives.

The second option involved in-depth thinking and multiple-step problems, and it allowed some room for alternate answers. The teacher reported that several students were quite excited about having a choice. Several were hesitant, not knowing which was the best test for them to show what they knew. Several had difficulty figuring out why the teacher might give partial credit for a wrong answer.

PORTFOLIOS

What Are They?

Portfolios are collections of student work for specific purposes based on criteria that support and provide evidence of application and understanding of the targeted concepts or skills. Portfolios can identify progress, show evidence of success, support evaluation and grading, and contain pieces that show what additional learning needs to take place. They are a way of facilitating ongoing feedback and reflection during the learning process.

An *e-portfolio* is a digital collection of student work where students can display assignments, work, projects, reports, and other documentation to show the way goals are accomplished. The learner can self-assess by correcting work while giving personal feedback and reflections. The teacher and peers also can provide specific feedback. Students can self-assess their work as well as make comments, to-do lists, and reflections.

Why Do We Use Them?

Richard Stiggins (1993) suggests that a portfolio is like a color video with sound, much more vivid than just a test paper. It gives a much fuller picture and provides supportive evidence to substantiate the feedback or grade that has been given. It also encourages student ownership and reflection on progress toward learning goals. Portfolios contain evidence of growth, with initial samples of work and pieces added periodically to show progress. Part of the portfolio process is the ongoing dialogue about quality and criteria that occurs between and among the teacher, students, and peers. This enables students to reflect on their work and to analyze quality and set goals.

How Do We Use Them?

Often, the portfolio is a partnership, with both the teacher and student being involved in selecting pieces to put in the portfolio. The teacher will set criteria for selection and allow several choices to be made by the student. Some teachers use colored dots to identify pieces that are included: red dot on student-selected pieces, yellow dot on teacher-selected pieces, and green dot on teacher/student-selected pieces. There can be four steps in the portfolio process: collect, select, reflect, and project (Burke, Fogarty, & Belgrad, 1994).

Collect

Pieces are gathered from the beginning of the year or unit based on criteria. They may include homework, projects, written pieces, mind maps, tests, assignments, videos, letters, graphic organizers, lab reports, poems, raps, audio files, and book reviews.

Evidence in the portfolio may be varied depending on the subject area.

Portfolios tell a story. . . . Put in anything that helps tell the story. (Paulson, Paulson, & Meyer, 1991, p. 60)

Select

Students select pieces based on guidelines. The criteria may include the following:

• Best piece/something I'm proud of
• Work in progress

- Student/teacher selection
- Most improved/difficult piece
- Special or free choice

Every so often, students will examine the pieces and decide which items should stay in the collection and which should be deleted. Pieces may be deleted for a variety of reasons:

- There is enough evidence of that competency already.
- It doesn't really show what is needed.
- A new piece is superior.

Reflect

Students will then write a reflection to be attached to the piece that explains why it was selected and what criteria it satisfies. Over time, students add other pieces that may show growth from the last item or can replace others. Not all pieces are necessarily the best effort, but may be included as baseline evidence to show growth in the future.

Project

Reflections and examination of items can lead to goal setting. Students can decide what to do next, what to focus on, what needs improvement, and what to celebrate.

Portfolio conferences are effective ways to share student growth with others. Students articulate their learning and goal setting to peers, parents, and significant others.

Each student is an individual, and each portfolio will be unique to each learner, showing the individuality and growth of the learner.

GRADING

Teachers give grades for many different reasons. There seems to be no commonly accepted yardstick for student achievement. Grades are often norm-referenced and subjective. But in this age of meeting the Common Core State Standards, grades should be criterion-referenced, based on standards for consistency and fairness, if they are used for ranking purposes. Opinions about what should be evaluated and what actually is evaluated are aspects of continuing dialogue among educators. Grades are often given for the following purposes:

- Measure content and skill mastery—to show what the student knows or can do in the subject area in a summative way.
- Chart progress—to communicate progress on individual goals and show the working level toward a learning goal.
- Motivate students—to prod the student to work harder or to reward the student for trying and giving so much effort. Many students are addicted to the reward of the grade.

- Provide information to a variety of audiences—students turn in their grades for recognition, awards, scholarships, and admittance into colleges and universities.

Grading processes need to be clear to students. Stiggins (2001) reminds us that students can hit any target that is clear, fair, and holds still long enough for all students to hit. Often the grade comes from a final test that is not criterion-referenced and not necessarily focused on measuring the standards. Rubrics and/or clear criteria must be shared at the beginning of the unit of study so that students know what to expect and work toward.

Often learning tasks and assignments are graded throughout the unit of study and averaged for a final grade. It seems unfair to grade at the beginning and throughout the learning process. Olympic athletes aren't graded before the final games; they are given corrective feedback related to how and what they are doing throughout the practice of skills and concept comprehension. Grading alone during the process would be of no help in fostering continuous growth to mastering the standard and is hardly faith, given that the knowledge and skills may be new and take some time for rehearsal and concept development. One bad day or absence could skew the final grade to an inaccurate representation. As Reeves (2000) points out, we should be treating assessments as physicals for diagnoses, not autopsies as finality.

If only a final test is given and graded, it may not be a true indication of students' knowledge and skill. They may have had a bad test day or been anxious about the test. Perhaps their reading ability prevented them from successfully answering the questions. Their limited comprehension of test terms may also have hindered their success. If the test was poorly worded and directions/questions too vague, this also could be a problem for the student showing his or her best, most accurate assessment of knowledge or skill. Culminating assessments such as projects, performances, and exhibitions are also valuable summative data. These allow students with different strengths and preferences to show what they know in a diverse and personal way. Rick Wormeli (2006) cautions us that fair isn't always equal and equal isn't always fair.

Grades (e.g., percentages, letter grades, ratings 1–4, pass/fail) are assigned for the final (summative) evaluation of what students have learned. Ongoing assessments have been giving feedback throughout the unit of study, and there are several possible class scenarios for the final evaluation:

- Give the common posttest to compare the pre- and postperformances. This is the same test given as the pre-assessment. The comparison of pre- and posttests may show progress or competence or lack of progress. If skills or content requires more practice, the teacher will need to plan for that to happen. The results could also show areas of weakness for further study. Posttests will determine whether students are knowledgeable, have improved, and have enduring understanding or need further practice for mastery to be acquired.
- Develop a test that evaluates the material studied by the different groups in the adjusted assignments. This test is based on the level of complexity of the study. Some of the questions would be on all tests. These questions would come from the information presented to the total group throughout the study. With this instrument, the groups of students would be given a written test

consisting of the material the individual groups had studied. This system allows teachers to communicate students' achievements on the specific information that they have been studying. They are not being compared with the students working on a less challenging or more difficult area of study.

- Some evaluation instruments combine both scenarios. There are questions given to all the students, and then a portion of the test is developed specifically to address an individual student or group of students.

All the above scenarios are examples of written tests given at the end of a section of study. They may not stand alone as a final grade. The written test grade may be only one piece of the data that compile the final grade. Evidence and grades have been gathered throughout to show a true picture of the student's performance.

FINAL GRADES

Many agendas influence the final grade. Some capable students do not work very hard but still receive an A. Other students apply themselves and work diligently to do their best but still do not get an A. Grades can motivate as well as show evidence of performance and acquired knowledge, but they also can be demoralizing. Comments need to be made that clarify the effort or lack of effort made by each student. When making written comments, write specific observable statements, omitting adjectives and adverbs. Just the facts! Adjectives and adverbs make the comments judgmental. Write down what you have observed in order to find patterns of behaviors, strengths, and weaknesses. This identifies specific needs for planning strategically. A strong work ethic is one of the competencies listed under "Self-Motivation" in Goleman's (1995) *Emotional Intelligence.* Teachers need to honor persistence, tenacity, and effort.

Tomlinson (2001) suggests that some teachers give students grades based on their success on the material they were studying. An identifying code can tell the parent that this grade was given at the student's level to show competency, not for comparison with the rest of the class. Thus a student might get an A working at his or her own level but a D in comparison with classmates.

As we move to a more differentiated classroom, we need to communicate with parents, students, and the broader community so that they understand our intentions and the changes that are taking place. When they comprehend, they will support the processes that are best for students.

As learning tasks need to be differentiated, so do assessment strategies, so that all learners get to learn in a variety of ways and show what they know in ways that are comfortable, durable, and suit the learner.

Chapter 4 Reflections

In your professional learning community, discuss the following, and share ideas and perspectives.

1. How do you currently pre-assess students?

2. How are you meeting the affective needs of your students? How do you incorporate the interests of your students into the learning experience? How do you combine these with prior knowledge and skills?

3. What data are you presently using to plan the instructional and assessment process?

4. What are you going to do first to improve assessment and feedback in your classroom?

5. Discuss feedback versus grading as a concept.

6. Are grading practices standardized and agreed upon in your school and/or grade level?

5

Adjusting, Compacting, and Grouping

WHEN WE DESIGN CLOTHES FOR PEOPLE, WE CONSIDER THEIR height, weight, and shape because those things influence the size of the clothing. As we know, not every student wears the same size, and of course we don't force them into a size small when they need a large. Not every student has the same background and experience, and so is not necessarily as knowledgeable or skillful in every topic or skill as other students. We also know that we may get tired of wearing the same old thing, and students get tired of the same old thing in the classroom, too. Yet we often force them to endure the same lesson (in the same format) whether they already know the content or haven't any idea what is going on. This is why adjustments need to be made in their learning. These adjustments do not always have to be responses to readiness but may be to suit interests and preferences as well.

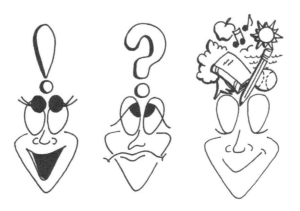

ADJUSTABLE ASSIGNMENTS

What Are They?

In classrooms everywhere, we are examining how we can get a better fit for all students. *Adjustable assignments* allow teachers to help students focus on essential skills and understanding key concepts, recognizing that they may be at different levels of readiness. Some may or may not be able to handle different levels of complexity or abstraction. Although the assignment is adjusted for different groups of learners, the standards, concepts, and content of each assignment have the same focus, and each student has the opportunity to develop essential skills and understanding at his or her appropriate level of challenge. The activities better ensure that students explore ideas at their levels, while building on prior knowledge and experiencing incremental growth.

Why Do We Use Them?

Using adjusted assignments allows students to begin learning where they are and to work on challenging and worthwhile tasks. If we were growing flowers and some of the seeds had sprouted and were ready to flower, we would not pull them out by the roots and make them start again from seed. It sounds a bit bizarre when we think about it. We, of course, would give the plants that were advanced in their growth the light, water, and food they needed and would nurture the seedlings that were just sprouting to help them bloom and grow. Adjusting assignments allows for reinforcement or extension of concepts based on student readiness, learning styles, and/or multiple intelligence preferences. Appropriate adjustments in the learning have a greater chance of providing a "flow" experience in which each student is presented with challenging work that just exceeds his or her skill level.

This also increases the chances of success for each learner because that success is within reach, and ultimately success will be highly motivating. Adjusting assignments also decreases the chances of "downshifting" and the sense of helplessness that students feel when a challenge is beyond their capabilities.

How Do We Use Them?

Initially, as in any planning process, the concepts, skills, and content that will be the focus of the activity are identified and aligned with targeted standards and expectations.

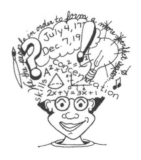

Using some method of formative pre-assessment (quizzes, journal entries, class discussions and data collection techniques, learning profiles, etc.), teachers gather data to determine the prior knowledge of students for the new content or the skill that is targeted for learning. The pre-assessment data are compiled. Then the key standards and concepts to be taught during the unit are determined. The teacher then decides which parts of the study should be taught to the total class and how they will be presented. The appropriate places to teach these concepts and/or skills are determined. Then comes the time to make decisions about any adjustable assignment. Assignments are adjusted to meet the needs of learners based on their present knowledge or skill levels. The following are questions the teacher will answer when making decisions about these assignments:

- What content does each group already know?
- What does each group need to learn?
- What strategies should be used to facilitate the learning of each portion?
- What is the most effective way to group students for each activity?
- What assessment tools will be used so that students will be accountable?
- Are the plans meeting the individual needs of the students?

Basic knowledge and experience vary among learners, so adjustable assignments may be needed. Here is an example that is typical of what teachers face every time they start planning for all of their students.

Example: Adjustable Assignments for Early Elementary Grades

The Money Unit

Figure 5.1, Part A, shows what the groups of students know and can do based on the pre-assessment data analysis. This does not show numbers in the group, but the knowledge or skill the group has. Part B is completed with tasks, assignments, or lessons that students require to continue their learning and understanding.

Figure 5.1. Adjustable-Assignments Model: Money

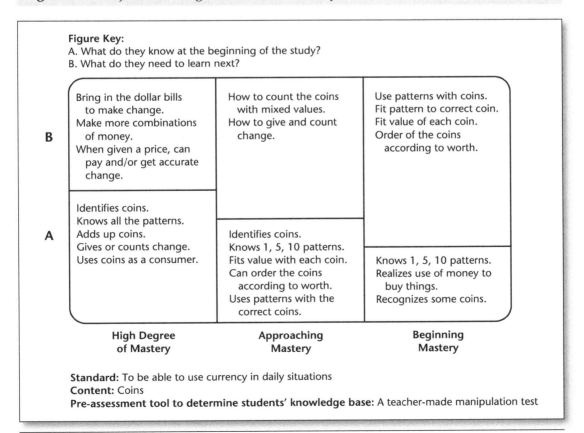

Figure Key:
A. What do they know at the beginning of the study?
B. What do they need to learn next?

	High Degree of Mastery	Approaching Mastery	Beginning Mastery
B	Bring in the dollar bills to make change. Make more combinations of money. When given a price, can pay and/or get accurate change.	How to count the coins with mixed values. How to give and count change.	Use patterns with coins. Fit pattern to correct coin. Fit value of each coin. Order of the coins according to worth.
A	Identifies coins. Knows all the patterns. Adds up coins. Gives or counts change. Uses coins as a consumer.	Identifies coins. Knows 1, 5, 10 patterns. Fits value with each coin. Can order the coins according to worth. Uses patterns with the correct coins.	Knows 1, 5, 10 patterns. Realizes use of money to buy things. Recognizes some coins.

Standard: To be able to use currency in daily situations
Content: Coins
Pre-assessment tool to determine students' knowledge base: A teacher-made manipulation test

Part A: High Degree of Mastery. What does this group know at the beginning of the study? Students know the names of the coins. They can count their money and make accurate change. They are consumer-wise as far as using money to purchase goods. Some of these students have been shopping in neighborhood stores. Therefore they have the background knowledge base. Other students will need those basics before they can proceed. Real-life experiences have taught the content. Therefore these students need to work with elements of money other than the basics.

Part A: Approaching Mastery. What does this group know at the beginning of the study? These students have shown that they know the names of the coins. They are limited as far as the other concepts being taught. Therefore they need to begin counting and adding up coins and working with different combinations of money. As they advance, they can move to purchasing and receiving or giving change.

Part A: Beginning Mastery. What does this group know at the beginning of the study? This group of students shows that they know few if any of the names of the coins or their worth. They will need all the information taught so that they develop a knowledge base.

Because of adjustable assignments, all these groups will be challenged and will learn information using a variety of strategies based on their needs. The students will work in groups that are designed to meet their needs. There will be ongoing assessment throughout the learning to provide appropriate feedback and to adjust assignments further.

Part B: Beginning Mastery. What do they need to learn next? From pre-assessment data, the teacher will be able to identify those students who have gaps in their previous learning or little background in the new area of study. Without filling in the gaps, the students will not be able to learn new information. During the study of the topic, allowances are made to work with these students where they are. The beginning group needs to learn the patterns that go with the different coins. For example, the students can count by fives but do not realize the same pattern applies to the nickel. In addition, the order of the coins by value needs to be learned. Many times, when children who are shown a nickel and a dime are asked, "Which is worth more?" many will choose the nickel because it is larger in size. The correct value has to be taught to be able to give and get change.

Part B: Approaching Mastery. What do they need to learn next? After a strong pre-assessment, the teacher may find there is a group of students who are ready for the standard content to be taught. Next they need to learn how to count the coins with mixed values and how to give and count change.

Part B: High Degree of Mastery. What do they need to learn next? When the pre-assessment data are compiled, there may be a group of students who know the content and will be bored if they have to go over all of it again. Although they know the content, they can always go deeper or be more analytical, creative, or practical with it. This group of students needs to explore different ways we are consumers. They also need to learn how to use more combinations of money, pay and get accurate change, and use dollar bills.

As a result of the information gathered during pre-assessment, the teacher designed three meaningful activities at the levels the three groups needed.

The more advanced group (High Degree of Mastery) worked at running a snack shop for recess and lunch. They priced the snacks and sold them, making change and counting the cash to calculate their earnings. They also used calculators to check their work.

During class time, these students engaged in activities that led them further in their understanding of coins and their relationships to each other. Using actual coins at a center, the students challenged one another with combinations. "I have ten coins that make a dollar," said Pat. "That's ten dimes," chimed in Tara. "I have six coins that make a dollar," said Corey. "That could be three quarters, two dimes, and a nickel," said Jodie. The game became quite competitive as pairs kept score of their successes.

Students also used calculators to total amounts of items on their wish lists for birthday gifts.

The group of students who were able to recognize the coins (Approaching Mastery) used coin stamps to make patterns with their partners. They challenged other group members to identify coins and give the total. They collected discarded toys and items from home and priced them to create a class garage sale. They priced the items and had a garage sale using money.

The group of students who needed more experience to recognize the coins (Beginning Mastery) played a coin game similar to Concentration, in which they had to be able to recognize the coins and match them. They also began to match equivalents, such as five pennies and a nickel equaling a dime, two nickels equaling a dime, and so on.

All students were able to shop at the snack shop and garage sale and practiced using coins appropriately. They also were integrated into the operation of the two sales and worked with more experienced students who modeled and added to their learning.

All students were engaged in interesting and challenging activities that added to their experience.

Figure 5.2 shows what the data might look like for a Spanish standard of everyday conversation and the topic of giving directions.

Section A shows what the three groups of students know and are able to do in relation to the standard and content. Section B would show what needs to be done to extend the learning for that group.

The **High Degree of Mastery** group (only four students) went online and found street maps of Mexico City. They wrote directions to areas or points of interest and produced posters advertising the attributes of that location.

The **Approaching Mastery** group designed a board game that used the vocabulary of giving directions. They produced interesting adaptations of board games with which they were familiar and wrote task cards for the games using vocabulary beyond what they had used in the past, incorporating new terminology.

The **Beginning Mastery** group worked in pairs to give one another directions to various areas in the school. They drew task cards and were able to direct one another to the cafeteria, office, or computer lab using Spanish. They then participated in a game similar to Twister, in which they spun a wheel and followed the directions given.

Figure 5.2 Adjustable Assignments: Spanish

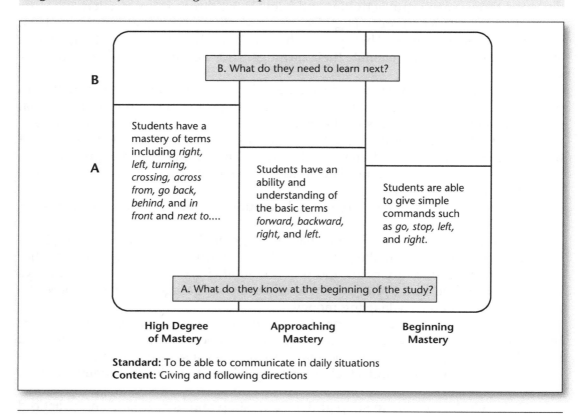

B. What do they need to learn next?

B

A

Students have a mastery of terms including *right, left, turning, crossing, across from, go back, behind,* and *in front* and *next to....*

Students have an ability and understanding of the basic terms *forward, backward, right,* and *left.*

Students are able to give simple commands such as *go, stop, left,* and *right.*

A. What do they know at the beginning of the study?

High Degree of Mastery   **Approaching Mastery**   **Beginning Mastery**

Standard: To be able to communicate in daily situations
Content: Giving and following directions

More levels of readiness may be identified and adjusted if needed, but when first beginning this process, three levels may be complicated enough for the teacher to manage.

After the pre-assessment has been given, the teacher analyzes the data and plots them on the chart in Section A (see Figure 5.3).

After the data have been entered, the teacher needs to consider what the students still need to know and be able to do to extend their learning. Teachers then fill in Part B of the grid with a learning that is suitably challenging and engaging in order to bring those learners to the next level. It may be a lesson, activity, task, or assignment. There may be different assignments that students do independently and that are given at two levels, in pairs, or in small groups, thus leaving the teacher free to interact and facilitate new content or processes with another group of students. The teacher may choose from a variety of curriculum approaches, such as projects, centers, integration, or problem-based learning.

ADJUSTABLE ASSIGNMENTS FOR TWO GROUPS

Students have been pre-assessed to find their knowledge base of an upcoming Common Core State Standard. The data is gathered and interpreted. Some students will be ready

Figure 5.3 Adjustable-Assignments Grid for Use by Teachers to Record Data About Student Readiness Levels

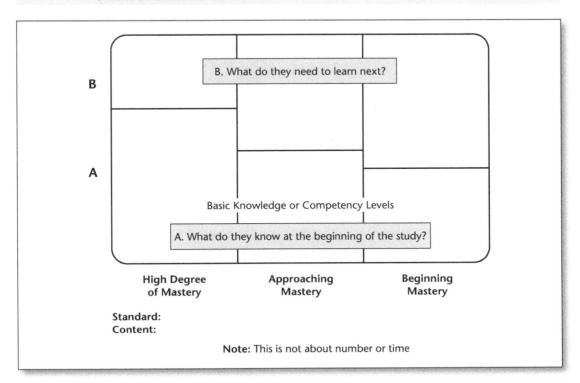

Figure 5.4. Two-Group Adjustable Assignment

Group A: Approaching Mastery	Group B: Beginning Level
Is ready to learn the new information. Has the proper background and is ready for the new material.	Needs to learn background information. Knows some but is not ready to work with the information being taught.

to learn the information because they have the proper background knowledge to learn the new material; for other students, determine if they have a gap in the learning that is necessary to acquire the information (see Figure 5.4). The teacher teaches the information. Now it is time for a student engagement assignment. Remember to plan both assignments so that they are equally stimulating, challenging, and interesting. Group A (Approaching Mastery) is assigned an assignment working with the grade-level standard that was just taught, and Group B (Beginning Mastery) is assigned an assignment to work on a gap that hampers the learning of the grade-level standard. These assignments are assigned simultaneously, so they should take equal amounts of time.

The following planner template, Figure 5.5, and Adjustable Assignment Grid, Figure 5.6, are used to plan for tiered assignments.

Figures 5.7–5.10 represent lessons in early elementary math and upper elementary science using the adjustable grid to design adjustable assignments.

Figure 5.5   The Six-Step Planning Model for Differentiated Learning: Template

Planning for Differentiated Learning	
1. STANDARDS: What should students know and be able to do?	Assessment tools for data collection: (logs, checklists, journals, agendas, observations, portfolios, rubrics, contracts)
Essential Questions:	
2. CONTENT: (concepts, vocabulary, facts) SKILLS:	
3. ACTIVATE: Focus Activity: Pre-assessment strategy Pre-assessment Prior knowledge & engaging the learners	• Quiz, test • Surveys • K-W-L • Journals • Arm gauge • Give me • Brainstorm • Concept formation • Thumb it
4. ACQUIRE: Total group or small groups	• Lecturette • Presentation • Demonstration • Jigsaw • Video • Field trip • Guest speaker • Text
5. Grouping Decisions: (TAPS, random, heterogeneous, homogeneous, interest, task, constructed) APPLY ADJUST	• Learning centers • Projects • Contracts • Compact/Enrichment • Problem based • Inquiry • Research • Independent study
6. ASSESS Diversity Honored (learning styles, multiple intelligences, personal interest, etc.)	• Quiz, test • Performance • Products • Presentation • Demonstration • Log, journal • Checklist • Portfolio • Rubric • Metacognition

Figure 5.6 Adjustable-Assignments Grid to Record Data About Student Readiness
Levels: Template

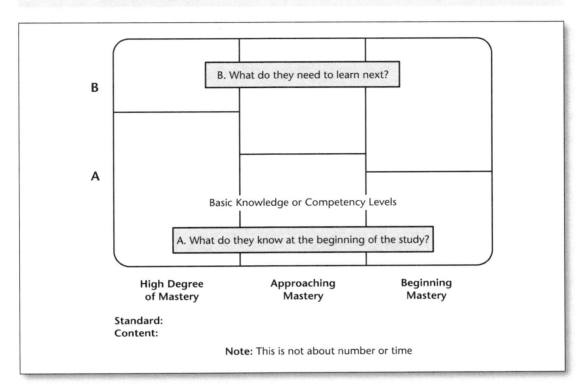

The lesson focused on early analog math also targets the following standards in the CCSS:

1. MD.3—Tell and write time in hours and half-hours using analog and digital clocks.

2. MD.7—Tell and write time from analog and digital clocks to the nearest five minutes, using a.m. and p.m.

The following standards are targeted in the next lesson focused on the periodic tables:

The student will investigate and understand that the placement of elements on the periodic table is a function of their atomic structure. The periodic table is a tool used for the investigations of

a. average atomic mass, mass number, and atomic number;

b. isotopes, half lives, and radioactive decay;

c. mass and charge characteristics of subatomic particles.

Figure 5.7 Planning for Differentiated Learning for Early Elementary Math: Reading the Analog Clock/Telling Time

Planning for Differentiated Learning	
1. **STANDARDS:** What should students know and be able to do? Read the clock to the minute. Count time using minutes. Count time using minutes and seconds. Learn how to read the clock for all times.	Assessment tools for data collection: (logs, checklists, journals, agendas, observations, portfolios, rubrics, contracts)
Essential Questions: What time is it?	
2. **CONTENT:** (concepts, vocabulary, facts) digital clock, hours, minutes, seconds, AM, PM	SKILLS: Reading the clock accurately in the same hour on most occasions. Reading the time on the digital clock when given a specific time and show it on the digital clock. Understanding a clock and how it works.
3. ACTIVATE: Focus Activity: Pre-assessment strategy Pre-assessment Prior knowledge & engaging the learners Label the minute and hour hands, seconds. Describe ½, ¼, and on the hour time. Name and discuss five important times in your daily schedule.	• Quiz, test • Surveys • K-W-L • Journals • Arm gauge • Give me • Brainstorm • Concept formation • Thumb it
4. ACQUIRE: Total group or small groups Use individual manipulative clocks to show various times. Partners explain how the hour and minute hands work. In a small group, have students brain storm about when they would need a digital clock so they are aware of the value of learning the skill. Small groups race to find the assigned accurate time on their manipulative clocks.	• Lecturette • Presentation • Demonstration • Jigsaw • Video • Field trip • Guest speaker • Text

5. Grouping Decisions: (TAPS, random, heterogeneous, homogeneous, interest, task, constructed)
APPLY
ADJUST
Beginning Mastery
Count by 5s with minute hand.
Learn location of each hand:
   on the hour
   quarter past, 15 minutes
   half hour, 30 minutes
   quarter 'til, 45 minutes
Approaching Mastery
Read the clock to the minute.
Count time using minutes.
Count time using minutes and seconds.
Learn how to read the clock for all times.
High Degree of Mastery
Needs opportunities to read the clock for all times automatically.
	• Learning centers
	• Projects
	• Contracts
	• Compact/Enrichment
	• Problem based
	• Inquiry
	• Research
	• Independent study

6. ASSESS Students will show the right time on the clockf aces when given a specific time. Test on the parts of the clock. Diversity Honored (learning styles, multiple intelligences, personal interest, etc.)	• Quiz, test • Performance • Products • Presentation • Demonstration • Log, journal • Checklist • Portfolio • Rubric • Metacognition

Figure 5.8 Adjustable-Assignments Grid for Early Elementary Math: Understanding the Clock and Elapsed Time

Standard, Concept, or Skill: Elapsed Time
Level: Upper Elementary
Key

A. What the learners know at the beginning of the study.
B. What the learners need to learn next.

B
Needs to read the clock for all times automatically.

Read the clock to the minute.
Count time using minutes.
Count time using minutes and seconds.
Learn how to read the clock for all times.

Count by 5s with minute hand.
The hour hand moves more slowly than the minute hand.
Learn location:
___O'clock: On the hour and location of each hand: quarter past, 5 minutes, half hour, 30 minutes, quarter 'til, 45 minutes.

A
Uses the clock daily. Explains how the hour and minute hands work.

Reads the clock accurately in the same hour on most occasions.

Tells time accurately on hour and half hour.
Recognizes time on clock of routines such as lunch time or dismissal time.
Understands and reads accurately elapsed time on the hour.

Reads a digital clock.
Can name parts of the clock: minute hand, hour hand
Knows 60 minutes is an hour.
Knows 12 numbers represent hours.

High Degree of Mastery   **Approaching Mastery**   **Beginning Mastery**

Figure 5.9 Planning for Differentiated Learning for Upper Elementary Science: Interpreting the Periodic Table

Planning for Differentiated Learning	
1. **STANDARDS:** What should students know and be able to do? Read and interpret the periodic table. Interpret charted data Learn each element and its location on the periodic table.	Assessment tools for data collection: (logs, checklists, journals, agendas, observations, portfolios, rubrics, contracts)
Essential Questions: What time is it? What does each element represent on the periodic table? What are the elements, and what do they mean?	
2. **CONTENT:** (concepts, vocabulary, facts) Element names and attributes of periodic table	SKILLS: Interpreting data and terminology. Learning how to read the periodic table. Learning how the periodic table is designed and its purpose Needs a thorough explanation of the process of working with the periodic table.
3. ACTIVATE: Focus Activity: Pre-assessment strategy Pre-assessment Prior knowledge & engaging the learners Can use a given key on the table. Locates and changes substance particles. Recognizes the periodic table. Learn the terminology. Use the key on the table. Learn the common elements and characteristics.	• Quiz, test • Surveys • K-W-L • Journals • Arm gauge • Give me • Brainstorm • Concept formation • Thumb it
4. ACQUIRE: Total group or small groups Interpret the data on the entries on the table. Determine number and mass by using the table accurately. Name reasons behind columns and rows. Name basic formulas using the table.	• Lecturette • Presentation • Demonstration • Jigsaw • Video • Field trip • Guest speaker • Text
5. Grouping Decisions: (TAPS, random, heterogeneous, homogeneous, interest, task, constructed) APPLY ADJUST **Beginning Mastery** Recognize the periodictable. Learn the terminology. Use the key on the table. Learn the common elements and characteristics. **Approaching Mastery** Learn how the periodic table is developed. Needs a thorough explanation of the process of working the periodic table. **High Degree of Mastery** Apply combinations of elements. Use the table with real-world problems and situations.	• Learning centers • Projects • Contracts • Compact/Enrichment • Problem based • Inquiry • Research • Independent study

6. ASSESS
    The definition and process of using the periodic table.
    Interpreting the table key.
    What does each entry stand for and mean?
    How does the table work?
    Who uses the periodic table, and when?
 	
Diversity Honored (learning styles, multiple intelligences, personal interest, etc.)
	• Quiz, test
	• Performance
	• Products
	• Presentation
	• Demonstration
	• Log, journal
	• Checklist
	• Portfolio
	• Rubric
	• Metacognition

Figure 5.10   Adjustable-Assignments Grid for Upper Elementary Science: Interpreting the Periodic Table

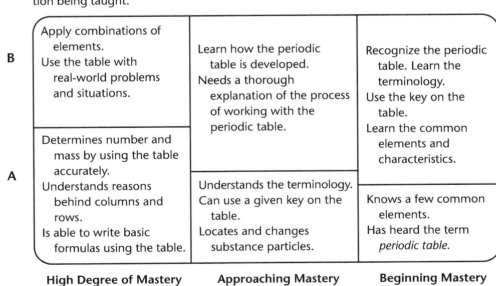

Standard, Concept, or Skill: Interpreting the Periodic Table

Key

A.   List specific knowledge base that the students know at the beginning of the study. This has been determined by a well-planned pre-assessment.

B.   To determine B, the teacher lists what each group of learners need to learn next. This challenges those who have a strong background at the high degree of mastery level, determines what those learners who are ready for the information need, and determines the gaps of those who do not have the basic knowledge needed to learn the information being taught.

B

Apply combinations of elements.
Use the table with real-world problems and situations.

Learn how the periodic table is developed.
Needs a thorough explanation of the process of working with the periodic table.

Recognize the periodic table. Learn the terminology.
Use the key on the table.
Learn the common elements and characteristics.

A

Determines number and mass by using the table accurately.
Understands reasons behind columns and rows.
Is able to write basic formulas using the table.

Understands the terminology.
Can use a given key on the table.
Locates and changes substance particles.

Knows a few common elements.
Has heard the term *periodic table.*

High Degree of Mastery   **Approaching Mastery**   **Beginning Mastery**

PS.4 The student will investigate and understand the organization and use of the periodic table of elements to obtain information. Key concepts include

  a. symbols, atomic number, atomic mass, chemical families (groups), and periods;

  b. classification of elements as metals, metalloids, and nonmetals; and

  c. simple compounds (formulas and the nature of bonding).

S 4.1 The student will plan and conduct investigations in which

  a. distinctions are made among observations, conclusions, inferences, and predictions;

  b. hypotheses are formulated based on cause-and-effect relationships.

RTI and Differentiation

The Individuals with Disabilities Education Act (IDEA) of 2004 suggested the use of Response to Intervention (RTI) to meet the diverse needs of students. The model consists of three levels, or tiers, of instructional practices based on the screening of students and early detection of gaps and interventions to help students who are struggling before they fall behind.

> The purpose of RtI is squarely improving results for students: All students. Indeed, RtI is not about special education, nor general education, nor talented and gifted, nor at-risk, nor migrant education. . . . RtI is about Every Education. (Tilly, 2009, p. 12)

Tier 1 is for all students in the general education classroom and should provide differentiation of instruction using research-based strategies to meet the diverse needs of students. In the general classroom the teacher considers time, content, and process and scaffolds the lessons as needed considering readiness.

Tier 2 comes through pre-assessments and universal screening that identifies struggling students. Then targeted areas of need are identified and research-based best practices are applied in small groups usually in the classroom three to five times a week until the students meet with success. This method of early interventions prevents many students from becoming candidates for special education referrals and keeps closing the gap for struggling students. It may also be raising the bar in terms of depth and complexity for gifted students.

Tier 3 is when more extensive interventions are designed for students who are not making progress in a reasonable timeframe with Tier 2 interventions and require more individualized attention.

Special education may be considered if students don't respond to the targeted interventions. Gifted students may need acceleration, mentoring, or compacting to meet their exceptional needs.

A PLANNING TOOL FOR INTERVENTION INSTRUCTION

Determine the common standards that are addressed during this unit of study. The learning progressions in the Common Core State Standards help teachers see what comes before and after their grade level so that they can appropriately plan with depth and complexity. Knowing what students have experienced in previous years is helpful in the process of designing learning experiences for the year. Target the areas of need by analyzing the assessment data. This identifies areas in which learners show need for reteaching and areas where there is a gap in the learning. It also reveals what the learners know before and during the learning. Identify which students have the same area of need. Now you know the area of need and the students who need the intervention. The next step is to determine the most effective time to get the small group together for the intervention. Then apply the following procedure for a quality intervention.

1. Group A: Grade-Level Group
   a. Assign an independent grade-level assignment(s) to this group of students, who do not need the intervention.
   b. Determine the time it will take for them to complete the work.

2. Group B: Intervention Group
   a. Gather the group with the teacher for the intervention instruction.
   b. Teach the needed skill, standard, concept, or process. Use only part of the determined time.
   c. Assign an independent assignment for each of these learners to work on the information that was just taught for the remainder of the time allotted. This allows each member of this group to work with the information that was just taught.

Note: The teacher is able to now move around to both groups, answering questions, probing for processing, and assessing students.

CURRICULUM COMPACTING

What Is It?

Curriculum compacting is a strategy first shared by Joe Renzulli of the University of Connecticut (see Reis & Renzulli, 1992; Tomlinson, 1999, 2001). It provides for the student who is very capable and knowledgeable in a particular topic in a subject area. It is a way of maximizing time for the more advanced learner.

Why Do We Use It?

Many students, because of prior experience, interests, and opportunities, may bring to the topic prior knowledge and skills that have been acquired over time. These may have been acquired through voracious reading, travel, and personal interest about a topic or from a mentor or role model who has had an influence on the learner. It is for these students that compacting may be used on occasion in order to enrich their curricula, enhance and stretch their thinking, and help them develop into more self-directed learners. In many classrooms, where teaching to the middle is the norm, some learners are bored as they "repeat history," and others are lost because they don't have the background or experience they need to understand or be able to do what is expected of them. Compacting/enriching (see Figure 5.11) may be used with learners identified as high-end or advanced based on a pre-assessment.

Figure 5.11 Curriculum Compacting: Used to Provide Enrichment for Advanced Learners Beyond the Regular Curriculum

Phase 1	Phase 2 Analyze data	Phase 3
Exploratory Phase	**Mastery:** skills, concepts What have they mastered?	**Advanced Level Challenges**
Pre-assessment: • Test • Conference • Portfolio conference	**Needs to Master:** What else do they need to know?	• Investigation • Problem-Based Learning • Service Learning • Project • Contract
To Find Out What the Learner • Knows • Needs to know • Wants to know	**How Will They Learn It?** • Gain with whole class • Independent study • Homework • Mentor/buddy in or out of school • On-line learning	**Opportunities for Successful Intelligence** Sternberg, 1996 • Analytical • Practical • Creative **Assessment**

It is important to allow all learners to move at their own pace, thus creating the "relaxed alertness" that Kohn suggests (as cited in R. N. Caine & Caine, 1997). Challenging experiences that are perceived as "doable" in a learning situation put students into a state of flow, thus engaging them at their levels of challenge and not frustrating or boring them by giving them too difficult or too easy a task.

How Do We Do It?

Phase 1

In this phase, after an exploratory session in which students are able to access prior knowledge and discuss their initial concepts and knowledge, a pre-assessment is given. This may be in the form of any or all of the following:

- A pretest
- A conference where the learner shares knowledge and understanding about the topic
- A portfolio presentation in which students show evidence of their comprehension and skill levels

Phase 2

After the pre-assessment, the teacher analyzes the data and identifies what the student already knows and has mastered and what the student still needs to learn. This additional knowledge or skill may be acquired by doing the following:

- Joining the total-class group for that concept or information
- Independent study
- Homework assignments
- Collaborating with a mentor or learning buddy in or outside school
- Online learning

Phase 3

Once the missing pieces have been added, the students may choose or be offered the following:

- An investigation or research project
- An ill-structured problem to solve
- A service-learning opportunity
- A project
- A negotiated contract
- A special assignment

These assignments facilitate the challenge of applying students' knowledge and skill in a practical and/or creative way. Robert Sternberg (1996), a noted psychologist, has defined *successful intelligence* as including the aspects of being analytical, practical, and creative, not just knowing.

A CLASSROOM IMPLEMENTATION IDEA

Each student selects his or her preferred intelligence: analytical, practical, or creative. This identifies the most important area of contribution he or she gives during a group discussion, special assignment, or project. The student then forms a working group with a member from each of the other intelligence areas. The triad will need a problem or project to solve. Because of the makeup of the group, all aspects of the problem will be addressed.

A practical application might be to create something that might be useful to society. It takes the information and skill to the "bottom line" level and demonstrates usefulness, shows development, and solves problems.

An analytical approach might be a critical thinking lens whereby students would evaluate, justify, and classify. People using this approach model the school process of explaining, outlining, and representing.

A creative task could allow students to innovate or invent. They could generate, produce, and improve on the skills or content learned.

Ideally all students could benefit from taking the new learning beyond recall with a practical, analytical, and creative approach if time permits or having a choice in which avenue they pursue. This allows them to enhance their understanding and

Figure 5.12   In-Class Compacting

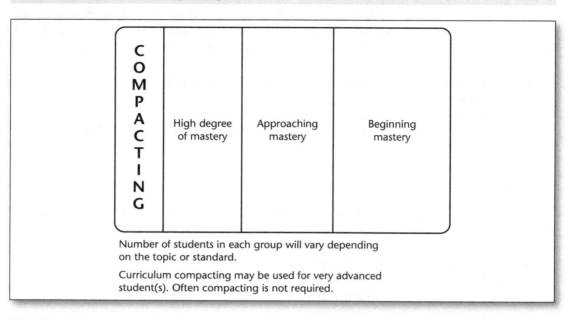

Number of students in each group will vary depending on the topic or standard.

Curriculum compacting may be used for very advanced student(s). Often compacting is not required.

also obtain an added perspective on the subject matter. Compacting/enrichment is a strategy often used with academically gifted or talented students to enhance their curricula. It may be done as a pullout or partial-pullout model or orchestrated in the classroom with the subject teacher. If students are pulled out, they should not miss other subject areas of study that they have not mastered. Teachers must be sure that students really do have full mastery of the concept, not just surface-level knowledge. Students should not be required to complete the regular classroom assignments in the subject for which they have compacted out.

What Does It Look Like?

Some forms of compacting/enrichment take into consideration that some students have ample prior knowledge or experience to warrant a full semester or grade-level subject advancement. This would include the French student skipping first-year French because she is fluent in the language. Another example is a pre-algebra student skipping Algebra 1 and starting in Algebra 2. Another scenario is the first grader going up to the third grade for reading each day.

Compacting/enrichment also occurs when students in several grade-level math classes are identified as being beyond curriculum expectations and so are pulled out of the classes during math time for enhanced or accelerated learning with an identified extension teacher.

In-Class Compacting/Enrichment

As shown in Figure 5.12, any class may divide into a number of groupings in relationship to mastery. There may be one or two, a few, or no students who need to have

Figure 5.13   Personal Agenda to Keep Track of Time and Tasks

❀ ❀ ❀   A Personal Agenda   ❀ ❀ ❀

My Agenda (name):   _____

Beginning on (date):   _____

Dates	Student Tasks	Log— How I Used My Time	Reflections	Completion Date— Teacher & Student Sign-Off

Figure 5.14   Double-Duty Log

Double-duty logs allow students to record or list facts and information about content or process and then reflect on that information immediately or at another time to integrate it into their thinking and deepen their understanding. It allows students to process the information and make sense or meaning. It also facilitates revisiting the material to clarify or add to the thinking.

Facts or Ideas	Thoughts and Reflections

enrichment offered because of a high level of mastery. The number of students in each group may vary depending on their skill levels in relationship to the standards.

We are not suggesting that you track students or restrict them to homogeneous groups such as the bluebirds, buzzards, and crows for any length of time. But sometimes skill development is needed at a challenging but not overwhelming level. This could be done occasionally to deepen skill levels and help all learners, beginning with where they are in relation to the targeted standard. Sometimes a small, homogeneous group will help students "drill deeply" with a skill, but more often, heterogeneous groups will be more helpful and allow students to "cross-pollinate" with a variety of fertile ideas.

Students may work alone, with a partner with similar interests, or in a small group focusing on the same materials and/or applications. This would depend on the number of students and their interests and learning profiles.

Agendas

The teacher may want to have students develop an *agenda* to keep track of time and tasks (see Figure 5.13). Students fill in the date and the task column of the agenda for the class, day, or unit of study. After each task is completed, they detail the progress in the log column and then chronicle their reflections in the next column. Each student and the teacher then conference and sign off in the last column.

Students may use double-duty logs (see Figure 5.14) to monitor steps and record reflections as they work on the assignment. This ongoing assessment helps both teacher and students clearly see the successes, progress, and needs throughout the assignment. It helps the students keep track of their time, reflect on their work, and set goals for the next step.

Adjusting and compacting are two techniques that strategic teachers use to help students feel comfortable and capable in their learning. Most instructional strategies can be used to adjust the learning.

FLEXIBLE GROUPING

Finding the Right Size

Flexible grouping is often needed to facilitate differentiated instruction. Everyone has strong and weak areas of ability and interest. Students need to be placed in groups that maximize their instructional time based on their performance levels. Grouping flexibility allows students to move according to their demonstrated performance, interests, and varied knowledge base levels. Students are grouped to meet their instructional, emotional, and personal needs. If a group of students get along socially, they will usually meet the instructional expectations.

By remembering to use each component of TAPS (total, alone, partner, small group) in planning, the individual social needs have a greater chance of being met. These grouping methods can be used where they fit in the classroom. Some students can work well in all of these ways, but every learner has preferences (Cherniss & Goleman, 2001).

A person who is very strong in his or her intrapersonal intelligence processes may prefer to solve problems better by working alone. He or she is able to solve the problem independently and does not see the need to work with a group. It takes time to think. Often this student will get really quiet in a group situation and become more metacognitive in order to process the learning.

Other students will be very strong in interpersonal intelligence. They are sometimes called "social butterflies." They feel the need to talk about concepts to understand them fully. They prefer to work with others rather than alone. These students bring empathy and harmony to the group.

Groups need the following:

- Ample space to work
- Clear directions and procedures
- Rules and guidelines established
- Individual roles assigned for group responsibilities
- A time frame assigned for on-task work
- To tap into all members' strengths

Some students learn best while working alone; some work better when grouped with others. This offers students options designed to tap into different readiness levels, interests, talents, and learning modalities. An effective, quality preassessment helps decide which type of grouping will be the most effective for that particular part of the learning. Flexible grouping is in constant use and is forever changing in planning differentiated instruction.

TAPS (a rap)

   Total Group

      Alone

         Partner

            Small Group

Remember!

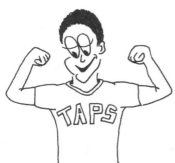

Some things need to be taught to the class as a whole.
There are certain things the Total Group should be told.

Working Alone, students get to problem solve in their own way.
They will be in charge of what they think, do, and say.

With a Partner, many thoughts and ideas they can share.
They can work and show each other the solutions there.

Effective Small Groups work together to cooperate.
Using the group's ideas and talents, their learning will accelerate.

So use a variety of ways to group students you see.
This TAPS into students' potential, as it should be.

Figure 5.15 lists definitions and some suggestions that might be used in each of the four types of grouping in TAPS.

Figure 5.15   TAPS Definitions and Suggestions

Total	Alone	Partner	Small Group
Definition			
Whole-class instruction All students doing the same thing Often teacher directed	Students working independently by choice or as directed	Students are paired through random selection (counting off, numbering, etc.) Teacher designed Students' choice Task or interest oriented	Random or structured by teacher or students Interest or task oriented Heterogeneous for cooperative groups Homogeneous for skill development
Suggested Strategies for Each Grouping			
Pre-assessment Modeling new skills Guest speaker Providing new information Viewing a video Using a small group Textbook(s) assignment Internet search	Pre-assessment Self-assessment Independent study Note taking and summarizing Reflection Journal entry Portfolio assessing Tickets out	Brainstorming Processing information Checking for understanding Peer editing Peer evaluation Researching Interest in similar topic Planning for homework Checking homework	Group projects Learning centers Consensus building Cooperative group learning tasks Problem solving Portfolio conferences Group investigation Carousel brainstorming Graffiti brainstorming

Source: Adapted from Gregory & Kuzmich (2004).

GROUPING STRATEGIES

The following are some ways to group students to better meet their learning needs.

Knowledge of a Subject

Cluster grouping of a small number of students in a heterogeneously grouped classroom can be used. This way, the students are grouped according to their prior experiences and knowledge about the topic. A pre-assessment is given to determine what the students know at the beginning of the study. This allows each group to be given tasks that involve a variety of opportunities for novices as well as experienced students. When grouped in this manner, students are challenged and are interested in the work rather than being bored by information they have already received or frustrated by something they know nothing about.

For instance, in a science curriculum, one or more students might be very knowledgeable about the unit on creatures of the sea. These students are a valuable resource to the entire class in this area of high interest. They need to study and add to their knowledge base rather than review the information they already know. The next unit studied in the science class might be something that is unfamiliar to them, so they would need to acquire the basics and move in with a different group to study. The knowledge base of an individual is based on experiences. The novice or beginner needs more of the basic topic information than the experienced learner does.

Ability to Perform a Task or a Skill

All people have certain talents and skills that they can perform better than others. One type of group to form would be the very skilled. Another might be those who are less skilled in a given area and need lots of help. Still another would be forming teams of masters, those who do the subject well, and apprentices, those who need one-on-one direction and assistance.

The purpose of ability grouping is for the student to work with materials and information that are challenging and stimulating at a personal level. Assignments differ by making adjustments consisting of varying levels of difficulty. Questions are molded to pull information from students according to what they can comprehend. This fosters continued growth because one size does not fit all.

Interests in a Specific Area of the Content

If a learner is interested in a topic or subject, the desire and emotions involved engage him or her. Conversations, interest surveys, and inventories give teachers information to weave into the learning. Why? By addressing what the learner is interested in, teachers have a link for the new learning. The desire to learn more is there. Students are interested in the arts, sports, games, role models, and outside activities that challenge their minds. In school, if their interests can be found, they are more likely to be engaged. Learning comes easier, and attention spans are longer for content that students are interested in learning.

Peer-to-Peer Tutoring

Having students assist each other with specific needs is a way to give them responsibility for understanding what they know and how they can use the information. The student who is tutoring is gaining from this experience. If you teach something, you remember it and realize what you know and how you know it. The learner is gaining from the experience, too, because it is individualized instruction that is tailored to a personal need. Students often communicate with each other using different words than the teacher would, and sometimes their ways of explaining information may be easier for the peer to understand. Some examples are peer tutoring, peer reading, and peer journaling.

A good time to use peer-to-peer tutoring is when a student has just caught on to a process, skill, concept, or standard. When the "lightbulb" goes on, learners want to tell others how they solved it or the details of their understanding. For example, a student has been struggling and working to understand a concept. She finally understands and "gets it." She is ready to tell everyone how this happened. She will give the step-by-step thinking process and explain it in language for others to understand. It is that "Finally, I got it!" feeling. There is a desire to say, "Let me tell you all about it!"

Automaticity happens through repetitive practice, and actions become hardwired in procedural memory in the cerebellum. This is the expert. It is a high-level thinking process to break down a procedure into clearly articulated steps. This reinforces the procedure in both the capable student and the novice.

Cooperative Learning

Productive and flexible partner and group work is essential in a differentiated classroom. Remember, if the people in a group get along socially, they will usually get the job done! Students learn social skills as well as cognitive skills and most often use higher levels of thinking as they discuss and clarify information.

When using cooperative learning:

- The group comes to a consensus on a common goal or a specific assignment.
- Those in the group are assigned specific roles to play for a particular task.
- Both individual and group accountability are built in as an important part of a cooperative learning experience.

Experts in cooperative group learning recommend that groups be structured heterogeneously:

> Of great importance to this discussion are the Lou and others (1996) findings that students of all ability levels benefit from ability grouping when compared with not grouping at all—students of low ability actually perform worse when they are placed [in] homogeneous groups with students of low ability—as opposed to students of low ability placed in heterogeneous groups. (Marzano, Pickering, & Pollack, 2001, p. 87)

Heterogeneity is more like how the real world works, where people don't necessarily choose with whom they will work. Thus in classrooms we need to give students the opportunity to work with others who have different interests, opinions, experiences, and abilities (Frey, Fisher, & Everlove, 2009).

The importance of *small groups* can't be overemphasized because if the group is too large, students may lose focus and the group has difficulty managing the process. Some students become "social loafers" and let others do the work. Sometimes a few students take control and eliminate the others. A large group is more likely to subdivide, with some students opting to work on their own.

Small groups, on the other hand, tend to increase the chances that everyone has a specific piece of the task and does it. The communication is optimal, and conflict is diminished.

For cooperative learning to flourish, students need to focus on developing and practicing social skills to greater increase the chances of successful interactions in group work. This is a 21st century skill that needs to be integrated into the curriculum for student success. Not only does cooperative group learning help social skills, it also increases student achievement and develops positive attitudes toward school and the discipline they are learning (Johnson & Johnson, 2009).

For heterogeneous groupings that occur randomly, try using the Stick Picks grid (see Figure 5.16), based on an idea shared by public school teacher W. Brenner (Fremont, CA).

More Heterogeneous Groupings

Differentiated instruction accommodates academic diversity and heterogeneous grouping. Wagon Wheel Teaming, based on an idea developed by Sheila Silversides (in Kagan, 1992), can be used to group students quickly and randomly into groups of three or four that include a beginning-level student, one or two average-level students, and an expert-level student. As shown in Figure 5.17, four concentric circles are fastened in the center with a paper fastener so that they can rotate. Students'

Figure 5.16 Stick Picks: Used to Create Random Groups of Heterogeneous Learners

By using sticks you can efficiently and quickly create random groups. As students enter the class, hand each one a stick. The following list shows you the colors to put on each stick. Number the sticks and use magic marker to put the two colors on the stick. You can use craft sticks or tongue depressers. After you group the students, collect the sticks so that they are not lost or destroyed.

Number	Color	Color	Number	Color	Color
1	blue	orange	19	yellow	orange
2	yellow	pink	20	green	purple
3	red	purple	21	red	pink
4	green	pink	22	blue	purple
5	yellow	orange	23	green	orange
6	blue	purple	24	yellow	pink
7	green	purple	25	blue	pink
8	red	pink	26	green	purple
9	red	orange	27	red	orange
10	green	orange	28	yellow	orange
11	blue	pink	29	yellow	pink
12	yellow	purple	30	green	purple
13	yellow	purple	31	blue	orange
14	red	orange	32	red	pink
15	green	pink	33	red	purple
16	blue	pink	34	yellow	purple
17	blue	purple	35	blue	pink
18	red	orange	36	green	orange

Every group of 4 sticks (1–4, 5–8, etc.) has all four colors: green, yellow, blue, and red, one on each stick. If that group of 4 is a team, then the teacher can assign the roles based on the four colors green, yellow, blue, and red. Random groups can be formed by partnering students with the same two colors. Some groups will have 2 students, some 3, and some 4.

To get 4 larger groups, use the colors yellow, green, red, and blue as group identifiers.
To form 3 large groups, use the colors orange, pink, and purple.
To get partners: 1 and 2 are a pair, 3 and 4, 5 and 6, and so on.

names are recorded inside the four circles based on readiness or capability relating to a particular skill or concept. Or student names can be assigned to a circle based on learning styles, multiple intelligences, or reading levels to encourage true diversity and heterogeneous groupings. To form a new student group, keep the center circle stationary, move the next wheel one turn, the following wheel two turns, and the outer wheel three turns. Then you will have totally new groups of four from the center to the outer edge, with all three types of learners in each new group.

Sharing Groups

Sometimes, teachers group students to share information, to research a topic, for review purposes, or to reflect and celebrate successes. Students can learn so much

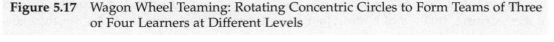

Figure 5.17 Wagon Wheel Teaming: Rotating Concentric Circles to Form Teams of Three or Four Learners at Different Levels

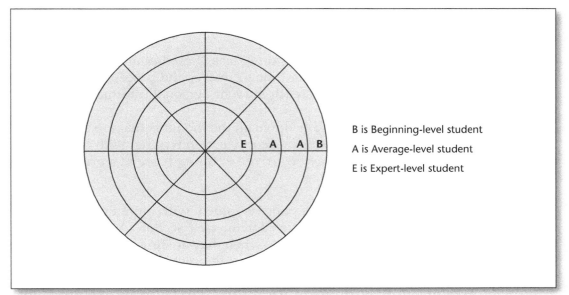

B is Beginning-level student

A is Average-level student

E is Expert-level student

from each other. It can be very refreshing for students to hear information from many sources, in many voices. It facilitates the opportunity for review and processing to reinforce and clarify ideas. It can also provide movement that is important to the physical needs of some learners.

Sharing can be done with students standing, sitting on the floor, sitting around a table, rearranging desks, or creating other comfortable spaces conducive to conversations. Plot these throughout the curriculum for conversations, discussions, and teaching that make the students responsible for their learning. This gives ownership!

Energizing Partners

Establish *energizing partners* for oral sharing and processing. Let students choose a classmate with whom they feel they can communicate effectively. For minimal movement, encourage students to choose a partner near where they sit. The partners leave their desks and stand and face each other to share information. Each set of partners decides who is Partner A and who is Partner B. This helps equalize talking time. The teacher assigns the task and assigns Partners A and B roles and tasks. For example, the teacher says, "Go stand and face your partner. Partner A, you share what you remember we discussed from yesterday. Now Partner B, you share what you remember from yesterday's learning." The established duo can remain partners for a length of time, such as a grading period, a semester, or during a particular unit of study. The reason they remain partners this long is so that the partners bond. They build trust and friendships and share information with more enthusiasm. However, in a differentiated environment, flexible grouping is ongoing, and all students need to and will work with all students at some point in time for a particular reason. This gives students a time to get out of their seats as well as to discuss the important parts of the learning. Instead of having just one student answer questions, half of the class is engaged in the learning at any given time.

Brainstorming Bash

Students form small groups and brainstorm ideas, thoughts, and solutions. After posing the task, give each group member time to answer and process the answer on his or her own. This think time gives each student personal information to share with the group.

Have a recorder in each group write down all the thoughts that are shared. This way, the group follows the conversation auditorily and in writing. With certain tasks assigned to the group, consensus may be arrived at through use of a brainstorming list.

Total-Class Brainstorming Bash. If the paper is folded, with more than one task to complete on the sheet, give the instruction for the first section. Assign a time for completion and a signal for the group to give when they are finished. Then go to the next set of instructions. This continues throughout the completion of the poster.

Adjustable-Assignment Brainstorming Bash. Give specific agenda sheets so that each small group can complete its brainstorming posters with the group's specific tasks.

Community Clusters

Community clusters use small groups to discuss strategies or to share personal thoughts, products, or facts. If the assignment calls for conversations, the teacher can decide the length of the conversation and can ask the students to stand in a "talking circle." Groups work best when they have no more than four students. If the students are sharing products or an artifact, they should form a circle at a table, on the floor, or at a desk cluster.

This group may be used for a variety of purposes:

- Share work findings
- Prepare a side of an issue for debate
- Process, reflect, and give input into the lesson
- Share personal information

Content Talk

Form small groups. Divide the assignment up, and let each group be in charge of reading, discussing, or preparing the assigned section with the total group. Assign roles so the responsibility is shared and the groups get the assignment done.

Research Probes

This assignment is given with a chosen or assigned topic to research. Students often need to come to consensus in their groups, choosing what they want to research. Then the desire to find out more about the topic is there. Encourage groups to divide up the assignment among group members.

For example, one student might go to the media center or resource center and look up the information. Another does a Web search, and another interviews and gathers information. Still another student might be the one they give all the found facts to and who records and organizes the data. Again this fosters evidence based reading using complex texts and resources as suggested in the Common Core State Standards.

Experiment, Lab, Center, Station, or Project Groups

Usually groups of two or three students form the most productive working teams. Sometimes this kind of group is used because of limited resources and materials, for example, technology equipment, media materials, lab supplies, or manipulatives. Students share information, work together, and produce a product, solve a problem, or learn new methods or processes.

Multiage Grouping

Groups are formed from students of different ages to learn from each other and work together. For instance, student groups of different age levels can work together with a common goal and learn. This establishes a potential mentoring situation or at least brings unique perspectives from the different age levels that interact with each other. This strategy is useful for reading, computer buddies, and problem-solving groups. Several teachers at different grade levels can facilitate the grouping of multiage students. Multiage grouping can also be used to enhance project work and investigation. The diversity of ages brings unique background experiences and knowledge to the tasks. Students learn from role models. Acquisition of language and creative ideas are often shared in these mixed groups.

Remember, tap into learning potential! Throughout their lives, students will need to work alone and with others. Learners need experiences in all group types to become effective working citizens in tomorrow's world. Teachers choose the type of group that is appropriate given the task, needs of the students, and targeted standards.

Adjusting, compacting, and grouping are important aspects of the differentiated classroom that meets a diverse audience with a curriculum that is more "sized to fit."

Chapter 5 Reflections

In your professional learning communities, discuss the following: Consider a unit of work that you will be teaching in the near future.

1. What are the expectations or standards to be taught?

2. What assessment tools could you use to get data about students' prior knowledge, skills, and interests related to these standards?

3. Complete an adjustable grid to represent the information acquired that is related to the content or skill.

4. What instructional decisions will you make responding to the data that you have organized?

5. What group work is integrated into your students' day, week?

6. Is there a balance of TAPS configurations?

7. Are these structures consciously constructed or randomly evolved?

6

Instructional Strategies for Student Success

J UST AS EACH LEARNER IS UNIQUE AND ONE SIZE DOESN'T FIT ALL, teachers realize that they need a wide repertoire of instructional strategies from which to pick and choose, adjust and modify. Taking a nip and tuck here and there in a garment is a beginning, but alterations are necessary if the garment is to fit comfortably and be wearable.

USING A VARIETY OF INSTRUCTIONAL STRATEGIES

Teachers need a vast amount of instructional strategies in order to teach information in a variety of ways. The key is to use the right strategy at the right time. Teachers are constantly gathering innovative ways to teach important information. Some favorite examples of these are visuals, graphic organizers, musical beats, mnemonics, processes, sequencing, seeking patterns, cubing, choice boards, and technology. Using stimulating hooks and intriguing closures with celebrations of successes are motivating strategies that entice learners.

After the information is taught, it is the student's time to be given an assignment to work with the material. Student engagement is the key! Vary the instructional strategies so that the learners never know what challenge they are going to encounter next. It takes personal ownership of the information for learning to happen. The instructional strategies and assignments must be timely, appropriate, and stimulating. Engagement is essential. One way to have success and motivate students is to give choices. The time is spent on an assignment that addresses the standard and is selected by the learner. Also, adjusting the assignment motivates a learner to complete a task because it is on a personal level of challenge and need.

BRAIN BASICS AND LEARNING

We know there are some things about the brain that are innate in all humans that impact how things operate in a classroom. Russian psychologist Lev Vygostky (1978) suggested a social development constructivist theory of learning on which many of the premises of differentiation are based.

1. Social interactions (teacher to student, student to student) foster learning.

2. To learn, one needs a more knowledgeable other (teacher, coach, or mentor).

3. Students will perform a task better and with more pleasure if the task is within reach and they have support from a more knowledgeable other. Understanding that every student is unique and has different "brain wiring" based on prior experience and background, the challenge must just exceed the skill level. This, Vygotsky suggests, is the *zone of proximal development.*

Pedagogy must be oriented not to the yesterday, but to the tomorrow of the child's development. Only then can it call to life in the process of education those processes of development which now lie in the zone of proximal development. (Vygotsky, 1993, pp. 251–252)

Although uniqueness is an issue, there are some things we know about how the brain works: It attends to new stimuli, processes information, and stores it in memory.

HOW THE BRAIN WORKS

Let us first examine the process so that we consider it as we think about differentiated instruction. One piece of vital information from brain research is that the brain continues to grow and thrive throughout life from external stimulation in the environment. Neural plasticity is the process of the brain growing and changing because of new learning opportunities. The brain actually grows dendrites (tree branch–like connections) between the neurons in response to environmental stimuli and multisensory enriched experiences (Diamond, 2001).

Brains change physically in classrooms where students are engaged in meaningful, stimulating experience and tasks. Information is taken into the brain by the senses; this usually is referred to as *sensory memory.* This is important for survival in the environment. It lasts for approximately three-fourths of a second.

Attention

The brain was put in our heads, not to go to school, but as a survival resource. Thus, the senses were the first line of defense to protect the species from extinction. Therefore all senses are on high alert for anything potentially dangerous or out of the ordinary.

Panksepp (1998) suggests all humans have a basic survival system. The brain hunts and searches for resources to exist. Exploring the environment is innate in all humans. The addictive behavior related to the Internet is an example of a 21st century *seeking system.* When we find what we seek, the medial forebrain bundle (the pleasure/reward center of the brain) is stimulated and triggers the dopaminergic pathway, releasing dopamine to create a natural feeling of euphoria. Success and enjoyment of learning can cause the same dopamine to be released. The seeking system may be one of the main brain systems that generate and sustain curiosity, even for intellectual pursuits (see www.youtube.com/watch?v=5smTLCKkUA4).

Of the five senses, visual, tactile, and auditory are the most efficient in capturing attention. There are many environmental factors constantly bombarding our sensory fields to capture our attention. Novelty, color, humor, and hands-on activity all grab the attention of the learner. Emotion also plays a large role in increasing attention. Positive or negative emotions may be the hook that generates attention or engagement. Strong negative "baggage," such as a bully in the schoolyard or a problem from home, may actually block the attention needed to focus on learning. When we are overstressed or overchallenged, the neocortex of the brain moves to the fight-or-flight mode and no thinking takes place. On the other hand, fun, laughter, play, and a high-challenge/low-threat environment help focus and maintain attention and raise the pleasure neurotransmitters such as dopamine and norepinephrine in the brain.

FOCUS ACTIVITIES

If teachers are going to capture students' attention, they need strategies to do so. Focus activities will do the following:

- Help the learner focus and pay attention
- Eliminate distracters
- Open "mental files"
- Provide choices
- Encourage self-directed learning
- Capitalize on "prime time"
- Fill unallocated time—extend, enrich, or "sponge" up extra time

Using focus activities or bell-ringers at the beginning of class helps students block out distracters, concentrate on activating prior knowledge, and sustain attention. Post the directions for the focus activity in a designated area so the students know where to find it when entering the classroom.

Anchor or Sponge Activities

Throughout the day, there may be times when students finish work early. The teacher can offer other tasks to "sponge" up the extra time without wasting instructional time. Tasks may also be provided for students to use as sponge activities when extra time is available. These tasks are also useful when the teacher is working with one group and students in other groups finish what they were doing. These sponge activities help students become more self-directed learners. Sometimes, students will focus on a personal quest or project that they are pursuing or some standard or skill that they are trying to master. Broader or more general tasks may be offered, such as the following:

- Develop a crossword puzzle on the computer to review the topic.
- Use the computer to develop a word web on this concept or topic.

- Revise your agenda for the week.
- Work on your culminating task for the unit.
- Use a word web to organize the ideas in this unit.
- Examine the items in your portfolio, and make some decisions regarding the pieces you have included. Should some be deleted or replaced at this point?

These more generic tasks may be posted for the week for all students to refer to when they have some time to sponge up productively.

Engagement activities should all be related to the objectives in the learning process, not just fun. They may be fun, but they should be focused on the necessary content or skills students should be developing.

Focus activities can take many forms. One teacher in a math class asked students to do the following with a paper and pencil:

- Pick a number from 1 to 9.
- Multiply it by 9.
- Add the two digits.
- Take away 5.
- Locate the corresponding letter in the alphabet.
- Pick a country that begins with that letter.
- Pick an animal that begins with the last letter of the country.
- Pick a color that begins with the last letter of your animal.

Then the teacher asked the students if they had an orange kangaroo in Denmark.

"Wow," they exclaimed. "How did you know that?" "You figure it out," she challenged them. They eagerly worked in pairs and analyzed the process and discovered that when you multiply any number by 9, the resulting two digits add up to 9. Then when you subtract 5 you get 4. The number 4 leads you to D. Under pressure, most people choose Denmark as a country. The last letter is K and *kangaroo* usually comes to mind. The last letter of *kangaroo* being O leads to the color orange. Then the teacher continued by reviewing the multiplication table for 9. This teacher knew how to make learning fun, add novelty to the learning, and challenge the students to solve a problem. The brain loves to make sense and seek patterns in information or processes.

In another classroom, the teacher had students begin the class by writing down on a small card or paper:

- Three things I learned yesterday . . .
- Two ideas that connected for me . . .
- One question I still have . . .

Here are a few other examples of focus or bell-ringer activities.

- Go on a scavenger hunt in your book and find _____.
- Solve the _____ problem on page _____.
- Go over your homework with a partner.
- Answer today's Brain Puzzle. (Post the puzzle.)
- Get the materials ready for today's activity. (List the instructions needed.)

K-W-L

Often, teachers use a K-W-L chart (Ogle, 1986). The K stands for what students already know about the topic. The W stands for what the students want to know. The L is used at the end of the lesson or unit of study to enable students to reflect on their learning and identify the information and processes learned.

This strategy opens up mental files to see what students already know and creates anticipation and curiosity about the new learning to come. It also brings closure and satisfaction at the end of the unit of study as they reflect on and articulate their learnings.

Other Strategies for Focusing

Other focus activities can take many forms, including challenges, questions and problems, or journal entries. Tasks may be offered that require recall and application of previously learned information. For example, students who read a chapter for homework can be asked to sit with a buddy and find as many "feeling" words as they can in the chapter that help develop the reader's understanding of the character.

Sometimes, teachers offer choices to students in order to capitalize on their interests and give them options. These techniques are also forms of pre-assessment that help the teacher and students set goals and design and select learning tasks appropriate to individuals or groups of learners.

The following example is a set of focus tasks that a teacher offered to students to allow them to make a choice.

From the chapter that you read last night, choose one of the following tasks and work alone or with a partner to complete it:

- Draw a comic strip to show the events in the chapter.
- In your journal, chronicle the events in the chapter.
- Describe the setting and how it related to the events in the chapter.
- If you were a newscaster, what would your progress report be?
- Rewrite a passage of the chapter in your own words. Use synonyms to replace some of the author's words.

Memory

Sensory input is either dumped out or passed on to short-term or working memory if the individual's attention is captured. Once attention takes data from the sensory memory to the short-term or working memory, the data are said to be *conscious*. The data last in conscious short-term memory up to 20 seconds unless we process them in some way.

We know that at the mental age of 15 years, the short-term working memory has the capacity for seven bits of information plus or minus two (Miller, 1956; Pascal-Leon, 1980). Capacity develops over the years, starting at age 5 with two spaces and increasing one space every other year until age 15. One way to deal with more than seven bits is to chunk them into larger pieces that hold more bits.

Rehearsal

Processing in working memory is often called *rehearsal*. Rehearsal or practice allows us to organize, analyze, make sense of, and remember the information. Rehearsal may be in one of two forms, *rote* (repeating information in the same form) or *elaborative* (connecting information with known data or embedding it in context; see Figure 6.1).

Elaborative rehearsal facilitates organizing and associating information into networks that are then stored in long-term (unconscious) memory. Rote memory may work for some learning, like multiplication facts that are drilled and memorized and put into automatic memory, but for enduring understanding (Wiggins & McTighe, 1998) to occur, students need more than "drill and kill."

Rote learning does not always have a very long shelf life because it has few hooks in the long-term memory. The brain is a pattern-seeking device and enjoys making meaning and connections between new ideas and those previously learned. Thus elaborative rehearsal strategies have a greater chance of producing long-term memories.

Figure 6.1   Rote and Elaborative Rehearsal

Rote rehearsal	Elaborative rehearsal
• Practice • Recitation • Drill • Repetition	• Mnemonics • Graphic organizers • Role-plays/simulations • Rhymes/raps/songs • Centers and projects • Multiple intelligences • Problems/inquiry • Performances • Exhibitions

Context

Context is an important contributor to memory and learning. A field trip to a farm or science center creates strong emotional hooks as well as enriched sensory stimulation. All these aspects will help solidify these experiences and concepts in the mind. *Episodic memory* is a term used to describe contextual or locale learning (O'Keefe & Nadel, 1978). It is processed through the hippocampus, as is *declarative memory*, which is concerned with the facts (who, what, where, when, and how).

Students often recall information better in the room in which they learned it. The context of the learning brings back vivid experiences of the learning that took place there. Students seem to do better on tests that are taken in the room in which they learned or studied. They also may do better on tests if the teacher who taught them is present in the room.

Emotions

Emotions play a large part not only in garnering attention but also in memory and learning. The amygdala, the brain's emotional sentinel (Goleman, 1995), imprints memory when experiences evoke strong emotions (LeDoux, 1996). Many key events in life and in schools are punctuated by and charged with emotions. For example, we all remember where we were when we heard about the 2011 demise of Osama bin Laden. The combination of context and emotion creates vivid memories.

Associating Concepts

One way to help students deal with massive amounts of content is to organize information around concepts. For example, students can organize networks of association under concept headings such as Change, Relationships, Persuasion, and Community. These mental concept files can be accessed, and a flood of information will be released as they are opened.

Concepts also help students see the bigger picture, organize the information, and deepen their understanding. Information is organized in networks of association throughout the neocortex and is unconscious until retrieved back to working memory.

When a "file of birthdays" is opened, for example, all the facts, thoughts, images, memories, and emotions dealing with birthdays come into conscious awareness. The neural network is searched and asked to recall all it remembers. One idea triggers another. This is why the process of brainstorming is a useful tool for activating prior knowledge. The brain scans the files, and one idea brings about another as the connections are revisited.

Recall and Rehearsal

Three things can occur after data have spent time in short-term memory. They may be dumped out (because they have no meaning for the learner or the learner wasn't given any practice to ensure that the connections between the brain cells grew enough dendrites), they may be practiced further, or they may be transferred to long-term memory. Once in long-term memory, the data can last forever, but if not used, they will become hard to retrieve over time (Pinker, 1998). "Use it or lose it" is true in this case.

Students often need many opportunities to recall and rehearse, many times and in many ways, in order to deepen their understanding. Doyle and Strauss (1976, p. 25) suggest that we give people too much gum to chew (content) and not enough time to chew it (process). Maybe what we need to retain valuable information is "less gum, more chewing," as suggested in workshops by Bob Garnstom, a well-known educator and organizational change consultant.

Retrieving information from long-term memory usually takes 3–5 seconds, depending on its quantity and complexity. This is why wait time (Rowe, 1988) is so important when asking questions. Because information is stored all over the neocortex in networks of association, it takes time to search those neural networks and bring long-term unconscious memory back to short-term conscious memory. Figure 6.2 shows progression of attention to short term and long term memory.

New information that captures sensory attention (sight, smell, touch, etc.) can be transferred to short-term conscious memory.

1. In short-term memory it can trigger the retrieval of other data.

2. When it is already stored in long-term conscious memory, in effect it opens closed files with previous information that was stored throughout the neocortex.

Figure 6.2 Learning and Remembering New Information: A Complex Process

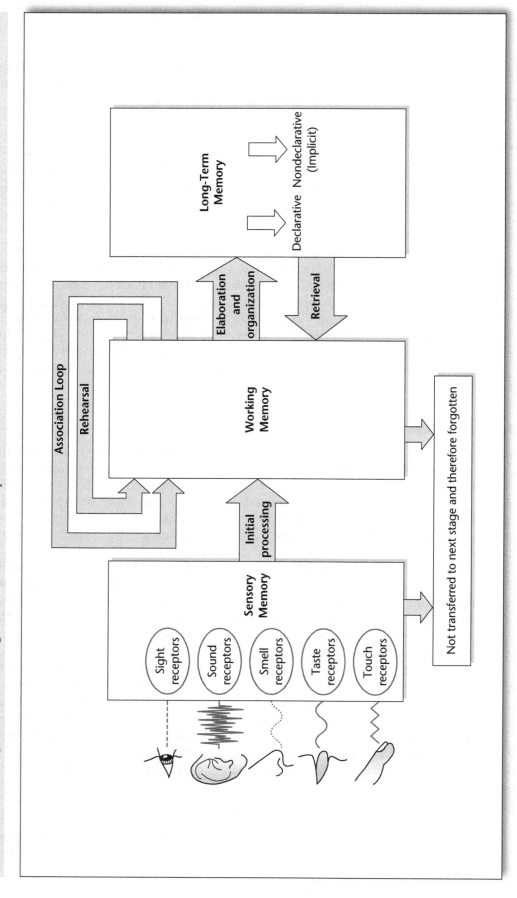

Source: From Nevills, P. & Wolfe, P. Building the Reading Brain, PreK–3, 2nd edition, p. 82. Copyright © 2009 Corwin Press.

3. By examining and relating the new data to previously learned data, the newer information can be transferred to long-term memory.

4. That is, it can be learned and remembered.

Long-term memory is really of two types: declarative and procedural.

Declarative	*Procedural*
The Facts • Who? • What? • Where? • Why? • When?	"Autopilot" (things one does without thinking) • Playing the piano • Riding a bicycle • Doing up buttons • Using the computer

Declarative memory is more conscious, whereas *procedural memory* is unconscious. Procedural memory starts as declarative. For example, when one learns to use a computer, each step is conscious and deliberate. Each step is in declarative memory: turn on switch, wait for screen, insert disk, double-click on icon. After many repetitions, the process becomes automatic and can be done unconsciously. These procedures are stored in the cerebellum (little brain). Students require lots of practice to send information and procedures to long-term memory. Practice may occur in numerous ways using a variety of multiple intelligences and as many modalities as possible to involve opportunities for visual, auditory, and tactile/kinesthetic learners to develop understanding.

PLANNING INSTRUCTIONAL STRATEGIES

Information about the process of memory is useful for teachers as they plan programs for a diverse group of students so that the students can realize their potential. Teachers may want to ask themselves the following questions as they plan:

- What do I want students to know or be able to do as a result of this learning experience?
- How will we judge success?
- What do they already know, and what are they able to do?
- How can attention be captured and sustained?
- What will the emotional hook be for the learners?
- How will new information and skills be acquired?
- How will students practice or rehearse to make meaning and understanding?
- How will they receive ongoing feedback during and after the learning?

REHEARSAL STRATEGIES

If teachers are to give students opportunities to rehearse in multiple ways they should pay attention to research based strategies for increasing student achievement (Dean, Hubbell, Pitler, & Stone, 2012).

Nine well-researched strategies hold promise for student success and interesting ways to interact with content and skills. They are divided into three groupings:

Creating the environment for learning

1. Setting objectives and providing feedback

2. Reinforcing effort and providing recognition

3. Cooperative learning

Helping students develop understanding

4. Questions, cues, and advance organizers

5. Nonlinguistic representations

6. Summarizing and note-taking

7. Assigning homework and providing practice

Helping students extend and apply knowledge

8. Identifying similarities and differences

9. Generating and testing hypotheses

Figure 6.3 shows the nine strategies with an explanation and information on what we know about the brain and how that knowledge supports the success of the strategies.

COOPERATIVE GROUP LEARNING

Cooperative group learning is one of the most researched instructional strategies in education today. We have gained valuable insight over the years from revered educators such as Aronson (1978); Bellanca and Fogarty (1991); Bennett, Rolheiser-Bennett, and Stevahn (1991); Cantelon (1991a, 1991b); Clarke, Wideman, and Eadie (1990); Dean et al. (2012); Johnson, Johnson, and Holubec (1998); and Kagan (1992). Working in cooperative groups, students learn valuable social skills, use higher-order thinking, and rehearse and practice new concepts, processes, and information. Cooperative group learning does not happen successfully unless it is well orchestrated and certain considerations prevail. These considerations increase the chances that the groups will work well together and achieve targeted standards (Johnson et al., 1998).

The acronym **TASK** (Robbins, Gregory, & Herndon, 2000) can be used to remember these aspects of cooperative group learning:

T   Thinking is built into the process.

A   Accountability is essential. Goal achievement: both individual and group.

S   Social skills lead to team success.

K   Keep everyone on TASK: roles, tasks, resources, novelty, simulations, and clear expectations.

Figure 6.3 Best Practice, Brain Research

Researched Best Practices	Brain Bits
1. Setting objectives and providing feedback • Clear instructional goals help students focus when the goals are stated in general terms and personalized by individual learners. Continuous feedback from the student, teachers, and peers is important.	The brain responds to high challenge and continues to strive based on feedback.
2. Reinforcing effort and providing recognition • The ability to relate effort and hard work to success • Growth mindset	The brain responds to challenge and not to threat. Emotions enhance learning.
3. Cooperative learning • One of the most effective and well-documented instructional strategies is the formation of heterogeneous groups to accomplish academic tasks. This strategy uses higher-order thinking skills and focuses on the development of social skills.	The brain is social. Collaboration facilitates understanding and higher-order thinking.
4. Questions, cues, and advance organizers • These help students open "mental files" to access prior knowledge before new learning takes place. This helps in pre-assessing the knowledge and skills (related to standards) that a student possesses and gives a context for the learning experience to come.	The brain responds to wholes and parts. All learners need to open "mental files" into which new learning can be hooked.
5. Nonlinguistic representations • A variety of methods, such as graphics, models, mental pictures, drawing, and movement, should be used to elaborate and rehearse new learning.	The brain is a parallel processor. Visual stimuli are recalled with 90% accuracy. The more areas of the brain that are involved, the better.
6. Summarizing and note-taking • The ability to summarize, delete, distill, and analyze information in order to be able to select what is important or relevant for learning.	The brain pays attention to meaningful information and deletes what is not relevant.
7. Assigning homework and providing practice • The ability to provide additional learning experiences that will help students further rehearse concepts and skills. Not necessarily more of the same.	The brain pays attention to meaningful information and deletes what is not relevant.
8. Identifying similarities and differences • The ability to classify in groups based on like attributes or the same theme or patterns can be explicitly demonstrated, supported, and encouraged. Compare and contrast.	The brain seeks patterns, connections, and relationships between and among prior and new learning.
9. Generating and testing hypotheses • This can be done through the inductive or deductive process. Students should be able to articulate their hypothesis and evaluate their accuracy.	The brain is curious and has an innate need to make meaning through patterns.

Thinking Is Built Into the Process

Cooperative group learning is ideal for embedding a variety of other instructional strategies that make a difference in student learning. Graphic organizers, thinking skills, and metaphors are easily used in cooperative group work to facilitate rehearsal and practice. Groups can be given tasks that are differentiated and adjusted to levels of the thinking taxonomy, a topic that we will discuss in detail later in this chapter. This will challenge groups at a variety of levels. Cubing, another topic we will discuss later in this chapter, also works well in cooperative group situations. Opportunities to explore content by using some or all of the multiple intelligences are possible. Students see many sides of a topic when using multiple intelligences as a lens.

Accountability Is Essential

Students who work together in cooperative groups generally produce a group product or project that is graded. Each student needs to be accountable for his or her personal contributions to the group and also for personal acquisition of knowledge and skills as a result of the group process. Teachers often use checklists or journal entries to collect data on the contributions and learning of individuals in the group. If teachers need to know what students know and have learned in the group session, individual tests, quizzes, demonstrations, exhibitions, and conferences will help clarify the understanding and competencies of each student. Cooperative group learning is a powerful strategy for learning, but we can't assume that everyone will know and understand the content and develop the skills just by being in a group.

Assessment may be multifaceted and include the following elements:

- An individual grade for the piece of work completed or the part of the presentation given
- A group grade for the final product or presentation
- A test or quiz on the content
- A mark for group participation

Consider the cooperative learning activity a learning experience. It is another way to blend individual needs with the learning, discussion, process, and investigation of the information. Then give an individual assessment to see what each learner knows about the information. This way, the work and the individual's grade are not dependent on the other group members. Group grades often cause problems and may create "social loafers."

Social Skills Lead to Team Success

Even though teachers work to build a positive climate and trust in the classroom, they may also need to teach social skills. Cooperative group learning not only helps students learn content and competencies but also helps them develop their emotional intelligence in the five domains (Goleman, 1995, 2006):

- Self-awareness: through reflection
- Self-motivation: developing persistence and a positive work ethic
- Managing emotions: learning strategies for conflict resolution and consensus building

- Empathy: listening, reflecting feelings, and behaving in a supportive manner
- Social skills: opportunities to identify practice and reflect on social skills

Students have different needs in these areas, and teachers will observe where those needs are as they monitor groups and recognize the strengths and weaknesses of their students.

Basic social skills that students need include these:

- Using appropriate language
- Speaking politely and quietly
- Encouraging others
- Listening to others
- Asking for help

Here are some social skills that students need to function well in a group:

- Disagreeing in an agreeable way
- Accepting different opinions
- Following procedures
- Checking for accuracy and understanding
- Dealing with conflict

Students need to know what a social skill "looks like, sounds like, and feels like" (Hill & Hancock, 1993) through conscious identification of the skill, modeling, practice, and feedback.

Teachers often post charts for reference that describe acceptable behavior in the classroom. Students need to contribute to the charts using their own language and terms. This increases clarity and ownership of the behavior and the probability that it will be practiced. Figure 6.4 is an example of a chart that describes listening to others. It was developed by a teacher and students during a conversation about the importance of listening to other people in a group.

Students then need to practice this skill with their groups and reflect on its use.

Individuals learn differently as a result of their experience and need a chance to contemplate their learning and their participation. Because students sometimes don't have the ability to reflect without guidelines, an organizer may be provided. Figure 6.5 is an example of student reflection after a group effort.

Figure 6.4 Social Skill: Listening to Others

Looks like	Sounds like	Feels like
Looking at the person	Tell me more . . .	I've been heard
Nodding and smiling	Mmm...	My ideas are valued

Figure 6.5   Reflection on Group Work

Date: _____

Name: _____

In my math class today we were involved in a cooperative learning activity.
This is a summary of what my group did.

My role was . . .

_____

_____

My behavior in that role was . . .

_____

_____

I helped achieve the group goal by . . .

_____

_____

I could have . . .

_____

_____

One thing I need to work on is . . .

_____

_____

Keeping Everyone on Task

Students in cooperative groups usually are assigned roles that increase the chances that they will work interdependently (Johnson et al., 1998; Johnson & Johnson, 2009). Roles such as encourager, clarifier, summarizer, or questioner can be assigned to keep the group functioning well. Other roles may include those that facilitate the task, such as recorder, reader, researcher, drawer, materials manager, or reporter. This encourages students to take responsibility and ownership for the task by assuming a particular role.

Some teachers may want to set up a scenario more like the real world and assign some of the following roles to students in a cooperative group (based on a workshop strategy by Kathy and Rob Bocchino, Heart of Change Consultants).

Production Manager. The production manager is responsible for the project. You will oversee and ensure that the other managers are working appropriately. You will manage the process, keep track of progress, and be the only person in the group who communicates with the CEO (teacher) when the group needs clarification or direction.

Information Manager. Your job is to ensure the accuracy and quality of the product. Your listening skills are valuable assets and help you make sure you clarify what the client is asking for. You will make sure all group members understand the client's/ CEO's expectations. You must adhere to any written directions.

Resource Manager. Your job is to gather and manage the materials necessary to complete the group project. Make sure all group papers and materials are properly stored away at the end of the period. If other objects, props, or materials are necessary, arrange to acquire them and make sure they are available when needed.

Personnel Manager. Your job is to manage the people on the team and build morale throughout the production. Encourage other team members, manage conflicts, and facilitate problem solving when necessary. Monitor for effort and productivity. Communicate any concerns to the production manager.

Technology Manager. Your job is to assist group members with all technical aspects of the production. You will help members with their computer skills when using the Internet for research, with spreadsheets and databases, word processing, presentation techniques, and troubleshooting.

Time Manager. Your job is to know when all deadlines are and remind others in the production team of those deadlines. You will keep a log of the steps and the progress. Communicate with the production manager concerning timelines and concerns. Communicate with the production manager concerning a particular team member who is not meeting time requirements. If more time is needed, ask the production manager to negotiate for more time.

The bookmarks in Figure 6.6 can be given to team members to help them keep focused on their duties for team success. Teachers may enlarge, photocopy, and laminate individual bookmarks for students' use.

Figure 6.6 Keeping Students on Task Bookmarks

Production Manager will:
- oversee the project
- ensure everyone does his or her job
- manage the process
- keep track of the project
- communicate with the teacher when group needs direction

Information Manager will:
- ensure accuracy of materials
- ensure quality of the product
- listen and make sure ideas are clear
- follow written directions

Resource Manager will:
- gather and manage materials
- properly store materials
- arrange and acquire materials and make sure materials are available

Personnel Manager will:
- manage people and build morale
- encourage team members
- help resolve conflicts
- help solve problems
- monitor effort and productivity

Technology Manager will:
- assist with technology aspects
- help with computer needs
- resources from Internet
- help with presentation techniques

Time Manager will:
- manage deadlines
- help team keep on track
- communicate with production manager
- negotiate time needed

Creating Interdependence and Building Alliances Within Groups

Teachers also can increase the interdependence in the groups by taking the following steps:

- Create a sequence to the process. Each group member has a role and a particular step to perform in the task.
- Provide limited resources (tools, texts, materials) that must be shared to complete the activity.
- Provide novelty and engaging scenarios or simulations in which students take on personas, such as investigator, researcher, or land developer. This creates a role that would be found in the real world and often adds authenticity to the activity.

There are many times when students work in cooperative groups of two, three, or four. In fact, working in pairs is a great way for students to build alliances in the classroom, by getting to work with many students to get to know them. It is also hard to get left out of a pair (Johnson et al., 1998). Partner work gives students a chance to practice social skills in a controlled environment with only one other personality at a time. It also builds community as students get to know one another one on one.

Whenever cooperative group learning is used as a vehicle for student learning, teachers need to ask the following questions to clarify the intention and process of the learning:

- What is it that students need to accomplish, and how will I communicate that? (Written task cards or charted directions should be clearly outlined for students so that expectations are clear and visible to all.)
- What will the size of the group be, considering the task?
- How will I group students, and why? (randomly, by ability, by background knowledge, heterogeneous but structured; see Figure 5.15, "Stick Picks," and Figure 5.16, "Wagon Wheel Teaming," in Chapter 5)
- What social skill will they practice and reflect on? (The social skill should be relevant to the task.)
- How will they learn about the social skill?
- How will they monitor its use?
- What are the timelines and guidelines for the task?
- What assessment will be used for the academic task? (presentation, product, report, performance, exhibition, test, quiz, etc.)
- What roles or tasks will group members be assigned to ensure interdependence and active participation?
- Are the groups functional?
- Do the groups get along socially?

Jigsaw

Another way to increase interdependence is by using a *jigsaw method.* Jigsaw (Aronson, 1978; Slavin, 1994; see Figure 6.7) is a very effective strategy, but not one that should be used with students until they have the social skills to deal with several members in a group as well as the skills to work independently. It is a powerful strategy for covering more material in less time. It enhances learning and increases retention. Students begin in a base group of three or four and are given letters, numbers, or names that will help them form expert groups. In the expert group, students are to access information or learn new material or skills that they will in turn teach to their base group. When they return to the base group, they teach their group members what they have learned.

Individual accountability is built into the process by having each member hand in a report, test, or quiz on the material learned or by calling on students randomly to report for their group.

The jigsaw method facilitates the sharing of responsibility for learning. It helps focus energy in a task and provides structure and process for the learning. It has inter- and intrapersonal components that also allow students to process information and move and interact with a variety of class members to gain a greater perspective on the knowledge or skills that are targeted for learning. It offers many chances for elaborative rehearsal and use of higher-order thinking through dialogue.

Jigsaws can be differentiated for students by giving them different materials and content to match different levels of readiness. Products, projects, or other authentic tasks and assessment that are expected from the group, based on their preferences and multiple intelligences, offer another way to differentiate.

The following example demonstrates how to build all the aspects of TASK into a jigsaw activity.

Figure 6.7 Jigsaw Strategy: Used to Enhance Interdependence With More Advanced Learners

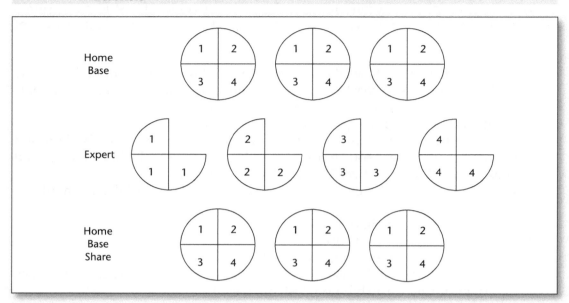

The Character Sketch (see Figure 6.8) is an organizer that can be used by a cooperative group of four people when reading a story or novel. Groups A and B focus on the same character (perhaps the main character), Groups C and D identify a different character, and so on. The base group (Persons 1, 2, 3, and 4) cuts the organizer on the broken line and distributes the four sections. Each person in Group A meets with the same-number partner from Group B (i.e., 1 with 1, 2 with 2, 3 with 3, and 4 with 4). They discuss an aspect of the character depending on the section of the organizer that they have. For example, two students may have the quadrant that says, "Looks like." They would find evidence in the story of what the character looks like and then write their conclusions in that segment of the quadrant. As they work together, the social skill they use would be to clarify information and listen to others' ideas. Each group of partners meets to complete their sections of the organizer: "Looks like," "Seems like," "Does," and "Sounds like." Then the base groups reconstitute and review all the evidence and conclusions that they made. From this information, the group writes a complete character sketch based on all the attributes collected.

The organizer can be reproduced on large chart paper to increase the space for collected information and to allow all participants to see the information. Each group member has an organizer to collect data personally from other expert team members.

There is interdependence built into this activity through shared resources and tasks. The students practice social skills as they work. They access information and use evidence to support their thinking, both worthy standards in any classroom.

This organizer can also be modified and used to divide tasks in other subject areas in a jigsaw process. Students could begin in a base group and examine four aspects of a country, such as food, peoples, geography, and origins (or in biology, they could focus on body systems, such as respiratory, digestive, nervous, and circulatory), in their expert groups and bring that information back to their base groups.

Jigsaw Variations

Table Jigsaw: Each group is responsible for a different topic or aspect and presents their findings to the rest of the class.

Simple Jigsaw: Each person in a small group (three or four students) is responsible for a piece of the assignment and resources the team.

Full Jigsaw: As described above, beginning with a base group, breaking out to expert groups, and then back to the base group to share.

Questions Often Asked About Cooperative Group Learning

What Is the Best Way to Group Students?

If a group of students get along socially, they usually get the job done. Occasionally let students choose partners or small groups. Group work is not always a social decision. Students also need to develop skills to work with a variety of personalities and perspectives. Alternate with random grouping and self-selected and teacher-constructed groups.

What Do You Do With the Student Who Does Not Want to Work in a Group?

An independent learner, who usually does not like group work, works better with a partner than a larger group. Remember, this student is learning important social skills when working with others. He or she does need some independent work time to process the cognitive learning.

What Is the Best-Sized Group?

Students working in groups of twos, threes, or fours are the most successful. When needing consensus, use groups of three to break the tie. Remember that the size of the group is also decided by the task to be completed. If the task is complex, more students may be needed. However, when students are developing skills for group work, smaller groups are better. It is hard to get left out of a pair. There is less social conflict and plenty to do. There is more "airtime" for each partner, and generally students stay on task.

NONLINGUISTIC REPRESENTATIONS: GRAPHIC ORGANIZERS

What Are They?

Graphic organizers are useful thinking tools that allow students to organize information and to see their thinking. They are visual/spatial, logical/mathematical tools that appeal to many learners for managing and organizing information. Graphic organizers give visual representations of facts/concepts and show the relationships between and among new facts and previous information. They are also used to plot

Figure 6.8 Character Sketch: Used as an Organizer by Four Students When Reading a Story or Novel

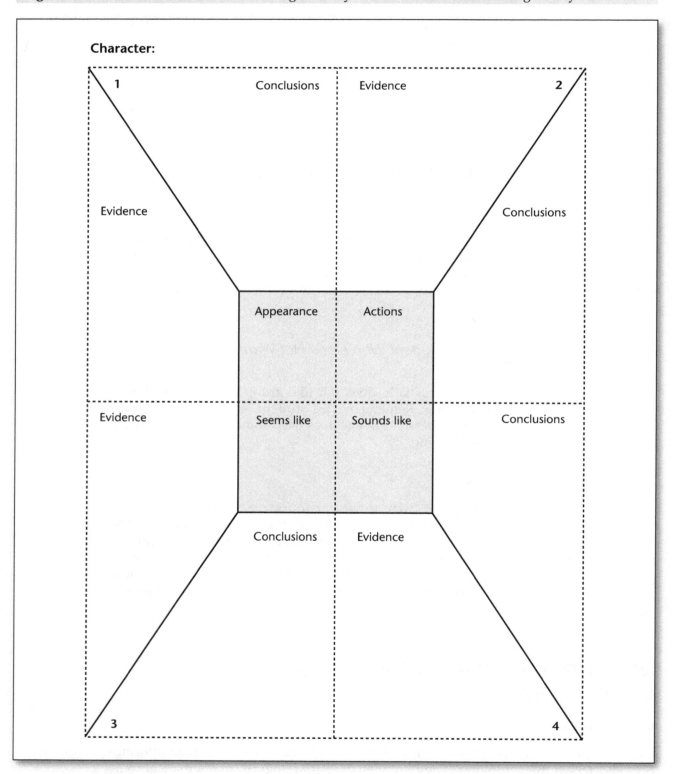

processes and procedures, and can be used at many points in the lesson. They may also be completed or designed online using sites such as Kidspiration.

WHY DO WE USE THEM?

The difference between good and poor learners is not the sheer quantity of what the good learner learns, but rather the good learner's ability to organize and use information (Smith, 1986). It takes time to process and pull random thoughts together. Sometimes a graphic organizer can be the answer to a difficult task. After learning the way to use the organizer, students are able to jot down their information their way.

Graphic organizers can be used in various ways:

- For brainstorming at the beginning of a lesson or unit to find out what students already know
- With reading assignments or when watching a video so that students can organize and capture information (The teacher may provide one, or students can design their own using the criteria given by the teacher, such as Who? What? Where? and Why?)
- To help chronicle a sequence of events or a process
- To relate new information to previously learned information
- To check for understanding
- For note-taking and summarizing
- For the culminating assessment

How Do We Use Them?

As with any tool, students need to be taught how to use the organizer and be given opportunities for practice with a full range of content and situations. Teachers model how the organizer can be used with content that is not too complicated. That way, students learn the process of using the organizer and can then use it with any content. Over time, students become familiar with the process of using a variety of graphic organizers. They will become adept at choosing appropriate organizers to fit the situation. Many students begin to design and create their own organizers to fit their needs. Using visual representations often appeals to the intrapersonal learner, who appreciates opportunities for processing and reflecting on new information independently. Organizers can be used independently, with a partner, or in a small group.

Effective Graphic Organizers for Comparing and Contrasting

Comparing, contrasting, classifying, and using metaphors are instructional strategies that increase student achievement (Dean et al., 2012; Marzano, Pickering, & Pollack, 2001). Students who spend time looking at the similarities and differences between two topics and perhaps plot these on a graphic organizer deepen their understanding and ability to use the knowledge.

Venn Diagram

The often-used Venn diagram (see Figure 6.9) identifies what is similar and what is different between two topics. A quick way to teach students to use the Venn is to have them compare themselves with a classmate in terms of personal characteristics, likes and dislikes, hobbies or sports, pets, and so on. They can brainstorm these characteristics individually and then plot them on the Venn with their partners, placing similarities in the overlapping center and differences on each side.

Comparison Matrix

A *comparison matrix* (see Figure 6.10) is another way to compare several items based on identified criteria. For example, when comparing states, the following could be listed in the left column: New York, Arizona, California, and Louisiana. Across the top, the following criteria could be considered: climate, population, geography, and size. This information, once plotted, can be transferred to a Venn diagram to identify the similarities and differences between two of the states.

Figure 6.9   Venn Diagram: Used to Identify an Area of Overlap Between Two Topics

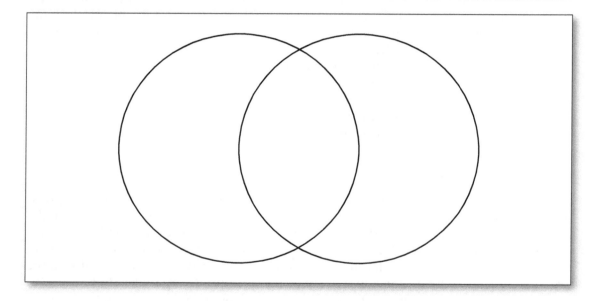

Comparing Two Things

Other forms of comparing and contrasting can be used. In Figure 6.11, any two things, ideas, concepts, or procedures may be scrutinized. At the top, in the first two frames, the two things being analyzed are put in place. In the two large boxes underneath, all their attributes are listed. Then all their similarities are selected and placed in the large frame underneath the Similarities heading. Finally, the ways in which the concepts differ are placed in the appropriate frames. Use the numbers so that the items in each box that differ correspond to one another. Students can compare forms of art, continents, scientific procedures, politicians, historical events, or any two pieces of content in any subject area.

Word Webs

The *word web* is an organizer that can be used for organizing and classifying. It enables students to focus on a concept, theme, or topic; identify the secondary categories related to the big idea; and then add all the significant dimensions related

Figure 6.10   Cross-Classification Compare and Contrast Matrix

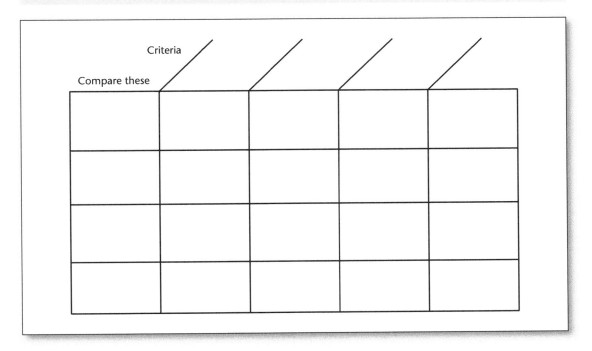

to those secondary categories. In Figure 6.12, for example, the big idea is World War II, and the secondary categories are the Axis, the Allies, Causes, Differences, Theaters of War, the Blitzkrieg, and Pivotal Events.

METAPHORICAL AND ANALOGOUS THINKING

Using metaphors and analogies is another way to show similarities and differences and to connect new information to more familiar objects or concepts. In Chapter 3, "Knowing the Learner," we used the objects beach ball, microscope, clipboard, and puppy to help clarify and understand the characteristics of the four styles of learning. By thinking of these four objects, students can easily recall the attributes of each one and in turn relate those characteristics to the four learning styles in order to understand them better.

Students can also relate new information by connecting it to something with which they are familiar. They may be able to understand the Renaissance if we ask them to explain how the Renaissance is like a video game, or understand the government if we ask them how the government is like an orchestra. When using two seemingly unrelated ideas or topics, we are causing students to examine comparisons and look at the similarities and differences between the two.

Having students stretch their thinking through metaphorical connections increases the likelihood of broadening their understanding of a concept or topic and remembering it in the future.

The quality of thinking, classifying, and deep understanding that it takes to create an intricate word web is a form of elaborative thinking and processing, as shown in Figure 6.13.

Figure 6.11 Comparing 2 Things Flow Chart

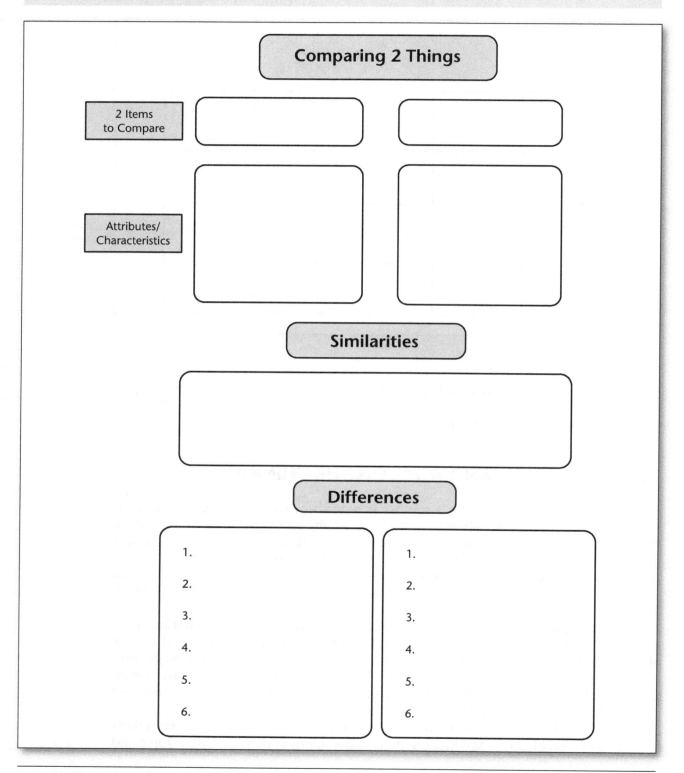

Figure 6.12   Example of a Word Web Used to Organize and Classify Primary and Secondary Concepts Related to World War II

A word web can be used to assess how well students have organized data. It also indicates that they have grasped the major concepts and made connections between them. It is also a useful tool to organize thinking in the prewriting stage.

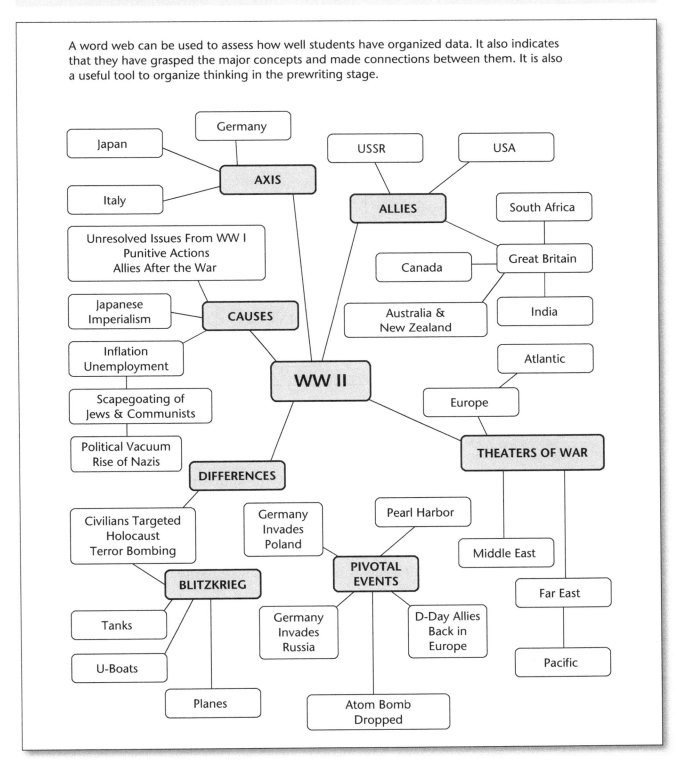

Source: Used with permission from Terence Parry.

Figure 6.13 Graphic Organizer Framework

Fact Frame	Roll It!	Inside Out!
Angle Antics	Star Connections	Drumming Up Details
Facts and Opinions	3 and 3	Summing It Up!

1. **Fact Frame:** Write fact in center box. Write supporting details in outer box.

2. **Roll It!** Write topic in the tire section. Write four key points in the spokes.

3. **Inside Out!** Write an important event, object, character, or place in the center. Write its attributes in the outer oval.

4. **Angle Antics:** Put a cause in each big triangle. Write the effects on each side of the cause.

5. **Star Connections:** Place the topic in the middle. Add a key fact in each star point.

6. **Drumming Up Details:** Write a prediction on the top of the drum. State the outcomes or learned facts on the side of the drum.

7. **Facts and Opinions:** Write the fact in the center. List an opinion by each arrow.

8. **3 and 3:** Write an important topic vocabulary noun in each of the large triangles. Write the meaning, a sentence, and draw a picture on the sidelines.

9. **Summing It Up!** In the top rectangle, write the fact. In the next two boxes, write two supporting details. Then write the summary or conclusion in the bottom figure.

ROLE-PLAYING

What Is It?

Role-playing is when a student takes on the role of a character, perhaps from a story, play, or novel; a historical or political figure; or someone depicting a particular scenario that deals with a concern or issue such as conflict resolution.

Why Do We Do It?

Role-playing allows students to process knowledge and demonstrate skills in an emotionally laden context. It is a form of elaborative rehearsal that causes students to interact with content and concepts and, ideally, create an episodic memory. It affords students the opportunity to examine and organize information, deal with issues, and create or re-create situations that have meaning. The roles students take on allow them to become immersed in situations. They become that person or character and take on that persona. As they play that role, their emotions are involved, and the emotional brain punctuates the moment. Role-playing allows students to be involved at their levels. Many students have strong verbal and interpersonal skills, and this technique allows them to use those skills. It also gives those bodily/kinesthetic students a chance for movement and expression.

How Do We Do It?

Allow students the opportunity to be involved when they are comfortable. Encourage students to choose the type of role-playing they would like to do. Try using a "choice board" similar to the one shown in Figure 6.14. Teachers find that they must work within the comfort zones of students; those who are more intrapersonal do not always embrace this technique because they may not be as gregarious as other students. Initially, teachers may have students engage in improvisation. As teachers begin to introduce this technique to students, they may want to use mime initially or provide a script. After several tries at role-playing, students may begin to write scripts for themselves. Props and scenery may be included if needed or available.

All students will need to identify appropriate audience interaction and behavior and monitor that behavior in role-playing situations. Feedback to participants should be positive and constructive. Reflection and emotional reactions should be processed after each attempt at role-playing. Role-playing places information and key concepts in a contextual learning situation and increases the chances for understanding and retention.

INDEPENDENT WORK ASSIGNMENTS

In every classroom, independent work is given daily. In a differentiated classroom, independent work time can be a time to meet individual gaps in the learning or challenge the students who know the information. Students are not always doing the same assignments. Some examples follow of activities that can be used as independent work assignments are listed on page 141.

Figure 6.14 Choice Board for Role-Playing

Format	Scenes	Props
Narrative actors	Transparencies	Artifacts
Interviews	Stage	Television frames
Mimes	Mural	Costumes

DIFFERENTIATING LEVELS OF THINKING AND QUESTIONING

Undue stress can occur during teacher-student question-and-answer sessions, and with excessive anxiety students can't access information filed in the neocortex. Fear of ridicule and inability to retrieve and recall occur when students are challenged by questions that are beyond their levels of understanding or comprehension. Wait time (Rowe, 1988) gives students time to access information stored in long-term memory. We know this takes at least 3 to 5 seconds. The quality or quantity of the answer is often increased by the amount of time given to access the information and formulate an answer. Generally, the longer the think time, the better the answer.

Think, Pair, Share (Lyman & McTighe, 1988) is a great technique to facilitate wait time. Asking students to think by themselves, pair with other students, and share their ideas naturally gives them time to think, access information, and formulate better answers. This also decreases the chances of overstressing students and increases the chances of them actually thinking about and attending to the question that has been posed. It encourages all students to share thinking, not just the person called on to answer. Studies show that greater retention and student achievement (up to 60% greater) will result when students are given more wait time for thinking (Black, Harrison, Lee, Marshall, & Wiliam, 2004). As the teacher comes to know the learners better and to recognize their levels of readiness, questions can be differentiated by level of complexity. This challenges learners at or just beyond their levels of comprehension or experience.

The following are samples of assignment activities for follow-ups after learning information by reading a passage or a teacher lecturette. Use these ideas to develop differentiated assignments, such as agendas, homework, centers, or projects, for the students to demonstrate what has been learned. These assignments also intensify the learners' knowledge about a standard, concept, or unit.

Record findings.	Discuss with a partner.
Hold a small group text talk.	Develop questions.
Write a song.	Create a rap.
Develop a cinquain.	Write a limerick.
Write a poem.	Write an advertisement.
Develop a collage.	Role-play.
Find the background music.	Portray a reenactment.
Develop a caricature.	Draw a picture.
Develop an editorial cartoon.	Make a diorama.
Write a cartoon strip with speech bubbles.	Color code.
Illustrate the ____.	Write the attributes.
Write adjectives or phrases to describe.	Create a timeline.
Develop a mural.	Design a new game.
Play *Who Wants to Be a Millionaire.*	Play *Jeopardy.*
Design a puppet.	Draw the setting.
Find the missing piece(s).	Draw a map.
Write an editorial with your point of view.	Use a manipulative.
Make a bar graph and interpret the data.	Design a brochure.
Create a pie chart and explain the results.	Scavenge for information.
Develop a key.	Prepare a point of view.
Act out the vocabulary words.	Name the causes.
Create a vocabulary game.	List the reasons.
List the synonyms or antonyms.	Write the main idea.
Write a summary.	Write the directions.
Develop a critique.	Draw a conclusion.
Write your opinion.	Write the fact(s).
Discover how it works.	Name examples.
Develop the sequence.	Debate the issue.
Invent a new way.	Identify the sounds.
Conduct an interview.	Write an ad.

Bloom's Revised Thinking Taxonomy

For years teachers have used Bloom's taxonomy of thinking skills to foster higher-order thinking skills in students. The revised taxonomy (Anderson & Krathwohl, 2001) broadens the opportunities for critical and creative thinking and includes the following skills:

1. **Remember:** Accessing long-term memory

2. **Understand:** Comprehending through words, pictures, and symbols

3. **Apply:** Ways to use

4. **Analyze:** Parts to whole

5. **Evaluate:** Make judgments using criteria

6. **Create:** Take beyond, rearrange, and innovate

Figure 6.15 Process Verbs for Thinking Skills

Thinking Skills	Process Verbs
Remember	List, remember, define, tell, state, label
Understand	Summarize, describe, discuss, locate, calculate, explain
Apply	Illustrate, demonstrate, dramatize, solve, apply, operate
Analyze	Compare, analyze, contrast, classify, question, experiment
Evaluate	Select, judge, evaluate, support, advocate, defend
Create	Invent, create, construct, design, develop, synthesize

Bloom's levels (see Figure 6.15) can also be used to layer the curriculum. In our lesson-planning template (see Figure 1.3 in Chapter 1), the levels of working with the content and skills include acquiring the knowledge or skills, applying and adjusting them in other situations, and assessing and evaluating their use.

Teachers may differentiate questions or layer curriculum based on students' readiness and levels of comprehension. Figures 6.16 and 6.17 offer samples of thinking level, definition, directing verbs, and question starters that may be used to align lessons and learning tasks with the different levels of the taxonomy.

We plan opportunities so that students interact with new knowledge and skills and develop an understanding and ability to retain and retrieve information in long-term memory. This is the learning process. By using verbs from Bloom's taxonomy, we can deepen understanding and learning using multiple rehearsals that "drill down" into the knowledge and skills. For example, related to a concept or skill, the Potential Activities column in Figure 6.17 can guide us to work through the "Acquire, Apply and Adjust, and Assess" process.

CUBING

What Is It?

Cubing is another technique that can help students think at different levels of the taxonomy (Cowan & Cowan, 1980). Cubing is a technique for considering a subject from six points of view (Cowan & Cowan, 1980; Tomlinson, 2001). It works well when we are locked into a particular way of thinking.

One side of the cube may say: Remember it.

Another side: Understand it.

The third side: Apply it.

The fourth side: Analyze it.

The fifth side: Evaluate it.

And the sixth side says: Create it.

Figure 6.16 Aligning Lesson Plans With the Six Levels of Bloom's Taxonomy

Lesson-Planning Steps	Thinking Level	Definition	Directing Verbs
Acquire	**Remember** Knowledge Learn information	Recall the facts and remember previously learned information.	Describe, list, identify, locate, label
Apply	**Understand** Comprehension information	Understand the meaning of and the how and why of events.	Explain, give examples, paraphrase, summarize
Adjust	**Apply** Use information	Transfer the skill or knowledge to another situation or setting. It tests knowledge and comprehension.	Infer, predict, deduce, adapt, modify, solve problems
Adjust	**Analysis** Examine parts	Break down information to specific parts so that the whole can be understood. Understanding structure can help with comparisons.	Discriminate, classify, categorize, subdivide, delineate
Adjust	**Evaluate** Judge the information	Combine elements to create new and different ideas or models.	Judge, compare, criticize, contrast, justify, conclude
Assess	**Create** Use differently	Rank or rate the value of information using a set of criteria.	Induce, create, compose, generalize, combine, rearrange, design, plan

Cubes may vary with tasks or commands that are appropriate to the level of readiness of the group. Cubes may also be constructed with tasks in a particular area of multiple intelligences, such as verbal/linguistic, bodily/kinesthetic, or intrapersonal intelligence.

Why Do We Use It?

Cubing, with its many sides, allows students to look at an issue or topic from a variety of angles and to develop a multidimensional perspective rather than a single one.

Figure 6.17 Question Starters and Classroom Activities Differentiated According to Bloom's Taxonomy

QUESTION STARTERS

Level I: REMEMBER (recall)

1. What is the definition for . . . ?
2. What happened after . . . ?
3. Recall the facts.
4. What were the characteristics of . . . ?
5. Which is true or false?
6. How many . . . ?
7. Who was the . . . ?
8. Tell in your own words.

Level II: UNDERSTAND

1. Why are these ideas similar?
2. In your own words retell the story of . . .
3. What do you think could happen?
4. How are these ideas different?
5. Explain what happened after.
6. What are some examples?
7. Can you provide a definition of . . . ?
8. Who was the key character?

Level III: APPLICATION (applying without understanding is not effective)

1. What is another instance of . . . ?
2. Demonstrate the way to . . .
3. Which one is most like . . . ?
4. What questions would you ask?
5. Which factors would you change?
6. Could this have happened in . . . ? Why or why not?
7. How would you organize these ideas?

POTENTIAL ACTIVITIES

1. Describe the . . .
2. Make a time line of events.
3. Make a facts chart.
4. Write a list of . . . steps in . . . facts about . . .
5. List all the people in the story.
6. Make a chart showing . . .
7. Make an acrostic.
8. Recite a poem.

1. Cut out or draw pictures to show an event.
2. Illustrate what you think the main idea was.
3. Make a cartoon strip showing the sequence of . . .
4. Write and perform a play based on the . . .
5. Compare this _____ with _____
6. Construct a model of . . .
7. Write a news report.
8. Prepare a flow chart to show the sequence . . .

1. Construct a model to demonstrate using it.
2. Make a display to illustrate one event.
3. Make a collection about . . .
4. Design a relief map to include relevant information about an event.
5. Scan a collection of photographs to illustrate a particular aspect of the study.
6. Create a mural to depict . . .

Figure 6.17 (Continued)

QUESTION STARTERS

POTENTIAL ACTIVITIES

Level IV: ANALYSIS

1. What are the component parts of . . . ?
2. What steps are important in the process of . . . ?
3. If . . . then . . .
4. What other conclusions can you reach about . . . that have not been mentioned?
5. The difference between the fact and the hypothesis is . . .
6. The solution would be to . . .
7. What is the relationship between . . . and . . . ?

1. Design a questionnaire about . . .
2. Conduct an investigation to produce . . .
3. Make a flow chart to show . . .
4. Construct a graph to show . . .
5. Put on a play about . . .
6. Review . . . in terms of identified criteria.
7. Prepare a report about the area of study.

Level V: EVALUATE

1. In your opinion . . .
2. Appraise the chances for . . .
3. Grade or rank the . . .
4. What do you think should be the outcome?
5. What solution do you favor and why?
6. Which systems are best? Worst?
7. Rate the relative value of these ideas to . . .
8. Which is the better bargain?

1. Prepare a list of criteria you would use to judge a . . . Indicate priority ratings you would give.
2. Conduct a debate about an issue.
3. Prepare an annotated bibliography . . .
4. Form a discussion panel on the topic of . . .
5. Prepare a case to present your opinions about . . .
6. List some common assumptions about . . . Rationalize your reactions.

Level VI: CREATE

1. Can you design a . . . ?
2. Why not compose a song about . . . ?
3. Why don't you devise your own way to . . . ?
4. Can you create new and unusual uses for . . . ?
5. Can you develop a proposal for . . . ?
6. How would you deal with . . . ?
7. Invent a scheme that would . . .

1. Create a model that shows your new ideas.
2. Devise an original plan or experiment for . . .
3. Finish the incomplete . . .
4. Make a hypothesis about . . .
5. Change . . . so that it will . . .
6. Propose a method to . . .
7. Prescribe a way to . . .
8. Give the book a new title.

Cubes offer a chance to differentiate learning by readiness (familiarity with content or level of skill), student interest, and/or learning profile (multiple intelligences). Cubes may vary in color and tasks depending on the abilities and interests of the small group. They add an element of novelty and fun to the learning by providing uniqueness to the lesson. It is a great strategy for tactile/kinesthetic learners as they reinforce understanding and extend or demonstrate learning.

How Do We Use It?

1. Keep clear learning goals in mind when considering the use of cubing for different learners.

2. Provide extended opportunities, materials, and learning situations that are appropriate for a wide range of readiness, interests, and learning styles.

3. Make sure students understand the verbs and directions for the tasks.

4. Group students according to readiness, with different colored cubes giving tasks or questions appropriate to their levels of understanding and ability in that particular topic or skill. Students assist one another in their learning.

5. Ask students to share findings with the large group or to form base groups of experts to share their tasks.

Figure 6.18 suggests verbs that may be used on all six sides of a cube.

Cubing may also be differentiated using multiple intelligences. Cubes may be designed with a variety of multiple intelligences activities to give students a chance to use their varied strengths. As an alternative, teachers can also use a die with numbers 1 to 6 and provide students with activity cards at various levels of complexity related to the topic (see Figure 6.19).

If students are studying the planets, for example, they might have a variety of cubes in the different multiple intelligences to process information for musical/rhythmic, bodily/kinesthetic, visual/spatial, naturalist, logical/mathematical, interpersonal, or intrapersonal intelligences. Or in a class where students are reading *Charlotte's Web*, by E. B. White, cubes could be used to deal with visual/spatial intelligence, and students could be given the following statements on the sides of their cubes.

Green Cube

1. Draw Charlotte as you think she looks.

2. Use a Venn diagram to compare Charlotte and Fern.

3. Use a comic strip to tell what happened in this chapter.

4. Shut your eyes and describe the barn. Jot down your ideas.

5. In your opinion, why is Charlotte a good friend?

6. Predict what will happen in the next chapter. Use symbols.

Figure 6.18 Use of Different Verbs, Tasks, and Commands on Each Side of a Cube

Cubing . . . Levels of Thinking

1. Tell
  Describe
  Recall
  Name
  Locate
  List
	4. Review
	  Discuss
	  Prepare
	  Diagram
	  Cartoon

2. Compare
  Contrast
  Example
  Explain
  Define
  Write
	5. Propose
	  Suggest
	  Finish
	  Prescribe
	  Devise

3. Connect
  Make
  Design
  Produce
  Develop
	6. Debate
	  Formu late
	  Choose
	  Support
	  In your opinion . . .

Yellow Cube

1. Use a graphics program on the computer to create a character web for Wilbur.

2. Use symbols on a Venn diagram to compare Wilbur and Charlotte.

3. Use a storyboard to show the progress of the plot to this point.

4. Draw the farm and label the items, people, and buildings.

5. When you think of the title, do you agree or disagree that it is a good choice? Why or why not?

6. What is the message that you think the writer wants people to remember? Draw a symbol that illustrates your idea.

Both cubes are tapping into using visual/spatial intelligence; the green cube is working at a more basic level, with key aspects of the story, and the yellow cube is stretching student thinking more in the abstraction, extending ideas and making connections.

Figure 6.19 Cubes Vary in Color and Tasks Depending on the Prior Knowledge and Interests of the Learners

Green Cube	Blue Cube
1.	1.
2.	2.
3.	3.
4.	4.
5.	5.
6.	6.

Yellow Cube	Red Cube
1.	1.
2.	2.
3.	3.
4.	4.
5.	5.
6.	6.

Teachers who use a variety of instructional strategies add novelty, choice, and individuality to the learning. These strategies allow diverse learners to find a size that fits and suits and to engage in practice and rehearsal to deepen understanding through as many learning styles and multiple intelligences as they can.

USING TECHNOLOGY IN THE DIFFERENTIATED CLASSROOM

Technology is a must in classrooms today. We are dealing with *digital natives* after all. Students understand it as part of their world and are motivated to readily use technological tools. Most classrooms have document readers, an interactive board, and a teacher's computer to use with the board. For many years computer labs have been common in schools. Today many schools supply computers for students to use in a station to share or tablets or laptops for each class member. This is an expensive endeavor but is proving to be well worth the investment. Other schools have mobile computer carts with enough tablets for each student. This means that the lab is rolled into the classroom and can be shared by classes at different times of the day.

Successful use of technology in the classroom depends on the knowledge of the teacher. There must be professional development training for teachers so that as the equipment is made available they know how to use it and make the equipment a working instructional strategy.

The positive aspects of using gadgets outweigh the negative, but there are some problems that can occur without careful monitoring and planning. Time on task and using time to teach and learn are important. The following are some of the problems related to using technology:

- Interruptions from unexpected glitches with the equipment
- A game becoming the focus instead of the learning of information
- Overuse that causes learners to get out of the habit of using other quality ways to think and solve problems
- Off-task behavior
- Misuse of the gadget

There are many opportunities for students to learn and practice on the computer so that they use higher-order thinking skills and problem solve. Instead of technology becoming the instructional tool or strategy, it needs to be one of many ways to teach. Memorable learning often happens when using technology to make personal links and connections to the topic. These can include a related video clip, music of the students' generation, or a web picture of something unfamiliar. Students can interact and exchange information with others from different parts of the world, other schools, and other classrooms.

Classroom response clickers get each student answering a question. Each member of the class, pair, or small group is assigned a clicker to respond to a posed question. The results are given so the teacher can assess opinions, misunderstandings, gaps in the learning, needs for interventions, or areas of mastery.

Technological gadgets are such popular items with students. The use has to be monitored and established rules enforced for successful use in the classroom. Clear expectations have to be established so as to avoid inappropriate use of gadgets.

More and more school districts are giving permission to use personal gadgets such as e-readers, cameras, tablets, and smartphones in the classroom. These gadgets are highly stimulating to the mind, and this concept is turning a recreational gadget into a useful learning tool. For example, smartphones are equipped to send text messages and emails, take and send photographs and videos, play games, and surf the

Internet. These are very useful and challenging during learning. Students often become bored with lectures and some assignments. They become excited and engaged if they are challenged to find answers and create unique ways of presenting information using their world of gadgets. The key is the teacher finding beneficial educational opportunities to use the gadgets at appropriate times. It requires constantly monitoring and enforcing the rules.

Less Paper and More Technology

More and more classroom teachers are planning lessons that use gadgets and computer programs for lessons, which requires less paper. For example, many projects are being done online. E-portfolios are being used as a way for students to digitally display their work, receive comments and feedback, self-assess their progress, and complete their goals. Classroom and homework assignments are being completed online as a way to communicate with peers as well as the teacher for feedback and assistance. Teachers are posting lesson plans, attendance, and having dialogue with other teachers, students, administrators, and parents online.

The success of this advancement means ongoing professional development for all school staff. They have to be trained in how to use the equipment and the programs. Also, it is vital to keep the equipment accessible, up to date, and working. Continually sharing new resources that are available provides the tools for successful classroom implementation.

Valuable Tools for Implementing Technology

Some of the web resources available are blogs, wikis, discussion boards, glossaries, RSS feeds, polls, surveys, social bookmarking, grading, lesson plans, and assignments (Chapman & Vagle, 2011). Continually search for websites to keep current with the most valuable tools for implementing technology in the classroom.

There are numerous instructional strategies, and we continue to learn and add to our expertise, like adding clothes to our wardrobes. However, as teachers build and increase their repertoires, they will see how they can adjust the learning for their group of learners and how different strategies appeal to different learners.

One size doesn't fit all, and, happily, one size doesn't have to.

Chapter 6 Reflections

In your professional learning communities, discuss the following:

1. Considering the Best Practice, Brain Research chart in Figure 6.3. Which strategies are you using on a routine basis?

2. Which instructional strategy will you incorporate into your repertoire in the next month?

3. How will you do that? With what content might you try it?

4. With whom could you work and plan for this implementation?

5. How will you monitor student improvement or reaction to the use of this strategy?

6. Brainstorm lists of focus activities and graphic organizers.

7. Design cubes for upcoming topics.

7

Curriculum Approaches for Differentiated Classrooms

NDIVIDUAL ITEMS OF CLOTHING ARE PUT TOGETHER TO FORM a wardrobe. Wardrobes evolve and build over time as we add and discard articles. A variety of instructional tools develop and, when used strategically, are powerful in a differentiated classroom. The tools can be built into various curriculum approaches. The curriculum can be delivered in many ways so it will appeal to individual learners and their needs for novelty, engaging activities, and quests for meaning. In this chapter, we explore centers, projects, choice boards, problem-based learning, inquiry and investigation, and academic contracts.

CENTERS

What Are They?

A *center* is a collection of material designed purposely with a goal in mind. Centers are very brain-friendly as they often give students choice, promote social interaction, and satisfy a wide variety of learning preferences and multiple intelligences. Centers can also be called *stations*.

Students work with center materials to develop, discover, create, and learn a task at their own pace. Students are responsible for their learning during center time. There is always an established purpose for each center.

The following are some valuable benefits for providing hands-on experiences in center learning opportunities.

- Remediate, enhance, or extend knowledge on a skill, concept, standard, or topic
- Pursue interests and explore the world of knowledge
- Work at their level of need and be challenged
- Be creative and critical problem solvers
- Make choices, establish their own pace, and build persistence
- Manipulate a variety of types of materials
- Facilitate complex thinking and dendritic growth

Centers are an ideal design for adjustable assignments. Centers can be set up in different ways:

- A variety of centers on a topic or theme in a particular subject area with different levels of difficulty
- Interest centers for further investigation of a topic
- Free-inventing centers for experimenting, discovering, and inventing
- Computer centers with multimedia resources for supplemental or remedial use
- Resource centers with a wide variety of reading materials
- Art media table to create artifacts that represent learning and creativity
- Role-playing centers to demonstrate characters and sequence of events
- Manipulatives centers for hands-on learning
- Skills centers for adjustable assignments
- Writing centers with a variety of writing tools and various types and sizes of paper
- Challenge centers for problem solving
- Listening centers with music or reading with both fictional and factual content
- Multiple intelligences centers that provide students with choices related to the topic

A structured center has specific tasks assigned and an agenda developed by the teacher. During center time, students work with skills or concepts, approaching them through a variety of experiences. Multilevel tasks are often designed for a certain skill or objective for this type of center. During center time, students work at their levels of need and at their own pace, while being challenged with complex, hands-on learning (Chapman & King, 2008).

An exploratory center provides materials and allows the student to decide what to do with those materials. For example, a reading nook is available with a wide variety of reading materials. The student decides which material to read and how long to read. A student settles down to read a selection because of a high interest in the topic and an appropriate reading level.

Establishing centers facilitates many diverse opportunities for learning to take place. The teacher can consciously adjust activities for the centers in the planning process and assign appropriate learners to the various centers. Centers are places where the work can be made to fit the learner's needs, ranging from basic learning, to remediation, to enrichment. They set up opportunities for understanding a skill or a concept through a variety of experiences. By having a variety of materials and tasks at one station, students become more responsible for their learning. They make their own choices and set individualized goals. There is an intrinsic reward for self-achievement. Centers provide opportunities to pursue individual interests and talents with greater immersion in the topic.

How Do We Use Them?

Choice Centers

Secondary history teacher Diane Huggler (Corning, NY) set up Ancient Civilization Learning Centers, which included the students' choices of China, Japan, Africa, the Middle East, Southwest Asia, and the Pacific.

The Goal. Your group's task is to discover as much about your civilization as you can from a variety of sources and present the information to the class.

The Procedure

- Each group has a set of color-coded folders that explain criteria for this task and help you discover information about your ancient peoples.
- Each person in the group will have a certain role in the group to make sure that it functions smoothly and completes its task successfully.
- Class time is to be used to complete the folder activities. Record your progress in the group log/journal.

The Presentation

- You will become the experts on your civilization and have the opportunity to share your knowledge with your classmates.
- Your group needs to prepare a PowerPoint presentation, with each group member being responsible for at least two slides.
- You may also use other teaching tools, such as the overhead projector, the chalkboard, maps, pictures, and so on, to tap the multiple intelligences.
- Your presentation needs to be at least 15 minutes long, and you need to be prepared to answer classmates' questions.

The Grade

- You will be assessed in three areas using a rubric that identifies how well you performed in the following categories:

1. Content

   2   4   6   8

2. Presentation

   2   4   6   8

3. Group skills

   2   4   6   8

4. Individual contributions

   2   4   6   8

Math Rotation Centers

Another scenario is the creation of Math Rotation Centers. Students work in each center to complete all tasks. They sign into centers the day before and keep track on their agendas.

Center 1. *Stock Update:* At this center, students are involved in a simulation of creating their own stock portfolios, such that they buy and sell stocks and keep track of the profits or losses.

Students are directed to complete the first update sheet in their stock folders, identifying profits or losses. They use information online or in the newspapers provided.

Center 2. *Folder Check:* At this center, students examine and organize their math portfolios. Portfolios should include notes, mental math papers, reflections, and mind maps of solutions, followed by all graded papers with corrections. Be sure the reflection is attached. When students finish their folders, they may move on to . . . the BIG ONE and Fraction Card Game: This center involves students playing games with others in groups with the same-color folders. The key concept is identifying equivalent fractions. Games may be played only after all players have completed their folder checks.

Center 3. *Changing Fractions to Decimals:* In this center students use Versa Tiles to self-correct activities. These tasks involve a basic understanding of finding equivalent fractions and decimals as well as an introduction to ratios.

Center 4. *Chocolate Delight:* At this center, students take an 8½ x 11 sheet of paper and fold it in half. After renaming the equivalent fractions, students are asked to write the explanation on the back half of the paper. Then they proceed to the self-correcting worksheets using a dry-erase marker, and they erase all answers when finished.

Differentiating Within a Center

When preparing differentiated activities for a center, it can be helpful to focus on standards to work with the three levels of the adjustable-assignments grid: *Beginning Mastery, Approaching Mastery,* and *High Degree of Mastery.* Depending on their mastery levels, students may be discovering, exploring, enhancing, or practicing the current information being taught; reviewing the information that has been taught; or exploring an upcoming topic.

Today's students play video and computer games that have many levels, so they are accustomed to this method. Center activity assignments can be color-coded and labeled, for example:

Beginning Mastery   Level 1: Green

Approaching Mastery   Level 2: Yellow

High Degree of Mastery   Level 3: Purple

When a student goes to the center, he or she first works on the area of need. After the assignment has been completed, the student can then work in an area of choice.

Thematic Centers: Experiments

The theme of these centers, adapted from versions used by the Halton Board of Education (Halton, Ontario, Canada), was Eggs. The centers consisted of scientific experiments that were part of an integrated unit called Great Eggspectations. In planning for two of the centers, teachers paid attention to the following:

- Standards and content
- Who will be working in the center
- Activities
- Materials needed
- Location
- Assessment
- Teacher reflections

Figure 7.1 shows a template that may be used to plan centers.

Management Techniques

Establish clearly defined, effective workspaces for centers. They might be a desktop, a carpet square, a lab station, a table, or a corner of the room. They are spaces for working with a particular set of materials related to particular tasks.

When setting up the centers, be sure to label the materials. For instance, if certain pieces go with one task, color-code or put a symbol on them to coordinate them as a set to enable quick identification. Also give them a "home" so they can be found and returned to the same location. This way, the materials are organized and labeled properly for easy access. Students need to assist in the distribution and cleaning up of materials. Design a system that is easy and efficient. Consider the uniqueness of the situation and plan accordingly. It is better to prethink management strategies than to have things go "off the rails" and thus waste valuable learning time while you rethink logistics.

Establish and teach rules so that all participants have a common understanding. Many times, the expectations for the regular classroom will also cover center work. For example, "Work quietly and respect others" is as relevant in centers as anywhere in the classroom.

Establish a common signal to get students' attention so all the students know what the signal is and what to do when they hear it. This is valuable when directions need to be given to a large group or when it is time to clean up.

Sometimes, students finish their work at a center before the time for center work is finished. That is when focus or sponge activities come into play. There should always be something meaningful and productive to do next. Often, it can be a reflection, journal, or log entry or another form of student self-assessment.

At times, the teacher is stationed in a center. Students rotate and come to the teacher's table to work. This works well when the teacher needs to give special attention to a particular group. The students at the other centers learn to self-monitor and become self-directed learners.

Figure 7.1   Center Planning Template

Center: Standards: _____ Content: _____ _____ _____ _____ Who: _____	
Activities	**Materials**
	Location
Assessment	**Teacher Reflections**

When centers have been set up based on interests or when students use them for sponge activities, they can eventually lose their appeal. At this point, the teacher should introduce a new interest center based on his or her observations and assessment of students' needs and preferences.

Students are often allowed to go to a new center of interest if time permits. Teacher monitoring and conferencing about quality work will mediate the decision to move on to a new center.

How Do We Assess Center Time?

One way to discover the thinking processes that students use when approaching tasks or problems is assessing center time. When asked the appropriate questions, students make their thinking known to the teacher. Assessment shows whether or where students have difficulties and which parts they understand and which need clarification. Proper assistance and follow-up can then be given to keep the students learning at their own rates toward the targeted standards.

Formative assessment during center time is essential. Students and teachers continue to dialogue, to give and receive feedback. Teachers who ask the right questions during this time can learn so much about their students. When open-ended questions are asked, students reflect on their thinking and explain their processes. Expressing orally how they solved that particular problem or accomplished a task enables students to become more metacognitive and reflective about their tasks. Using anecdotal note-taking or an observation checklist along with effective questions, teachers begin to understand where the students are in their learning/thinking and often where they need to go next. Assessment should inform practice and tell teachers how students are progressing and what adjustments should be made to a program.

Both the students and the teacher should pay attention to assessment data to inform the next steps.

Teacher Assessment Strategies

Teachers move in and out of the centers to interact with the learners and monitor their progress. Ongoing conferencing keeps learners on task and gives teachers the data necessary to adjust or change any activities that are not challenging enough or perhaps are too challenging. Ongoing modification is often necessary to adjust tasks when there is a need to do so.

Anecdotal Finding. Teachers often record anecdotal findings of observations for record-keeping purposes. Some teachers refer to this as "clipboard cruising." The data collection sheet may look something like the one in Figure 7.2, with columns for note-taking.

Checklists. Use a checklist to assess the behaviors being observed. Teachers observing center time design the most effective checklists because they are familiar with the information and its location on the list. It should take longer to develop the checklist than to score it. The teacher who will be using it designs the most effective checklist; each item fits a particular situation. Also, if the person who made the checklist is the one scoring it, he or she is familiar with the data and it is easy to use.

Figure 7.2 Clipboard Cruising for Data Collection

Clipboard Cruising

Name	Date	Time	Center or Task	Observed Behavior
_____	_____	_____	_____	_____
_____	_____	_____	_____	_____
_____	_____	_____	_____	_____
_____	_____	_____	_____	_____
_____	_____	_____	_____	_____
_____	_____	_____	_____	_____
_____	_____	_____	_____	_____

Center time checklists should address the targeted needs of the group. One list could address social skills; another, time cognitive skills; and yet another, both. Figure 7.3 offers some sample observable behaviors to include in a checklist.

Effective Questioning Techniques

Open-Ended Questions and Statements. Have students demonstrate what they know by asking appropriate questions. The right questions get students to convey their thinking processes, which are unique to how each student approaches a task or problem at a particular time. This evidence shows where there are weaknesses and strengths, misunderstandings or clarity.

The following are some examples of effective questions:

- Tell me what you are doing.
- How did you do that?
- Tell me step-by-step how you made that.

Student Self-Assessment

Students can use log and journal entries for self-assessment. Some suggestions for logs or journals include the following:

a. Today, I want to tell you _____. Choose one of the following that you would like to share:

- What I am doing
- Why I am doing it

Figure 7.3 Center Checklists: Used to Address Targeted Needs of the Group

Center Checklist

Name _____ Center _____ Unit of Study _____

Type of Assignment _____ Assigned _____ Student Choice _____

Teacher Date _____ Signature _____

Peer Date _____ Signature _____

Self Date _____ Signature _____

Work Habits	Not Yet	Sometimes	Most of the Time
Stays on task			
Gets work done on time			
Uses materials appropriately			
Completes tasks			
Follows rules at the center			
Uses time wisely			
Social Skills			
Shares materials			
Listens to others			
Helps others			
Respects self and others			
Shows patience			
Group work			
Takes turns			
Shares materials and ideas			
Participates appropriately			
Focuses on one person talking			
Communicates appropriately			
Works well with others			
Helps others			

COMMENTS:

- Why it is important
- How I can use it
- Why I chose to do this
- What I need next

b. Four Thoughts Feedback

- The part I like best is _____.
- The part I am not clear about is _____.
- Someone needs to tell me more about _____.
- Next time, I need to _____.

c. Today, I will receive the _____ award. Make an award certificate or ribbon.

Centers can be assessed by students independently after they have worked in them. Cards may be placed at the centers for students to give their feedback to the teacher. You may want to include some or all of the information in Figure 7.4.

Journal entries are also useful after center work. Here are a few suggestions for journal stems that help students reflect on their work:

- The best thing about this center time was _____.
- The worst thing about this center time was _____.

Figure 7.4 Sample Feedback Card for Students to Assess Centers After They Have Worked in Them

Name _____ Center _____ Date _____

At this center I learned _____

_____

_____

Centers that I worked in today were

1. _____

2. _____

While I was there I _____

How would you rate your learning?

1   2   3   4   5   Wow

- Next time, I _____.
- I learned _____.
- This is what I did, step-by-step: _____.

Center time can be some of the most productive time in the classroom. When the centers are set up with thoughtful, challenging materials focused on clear standards that develop students' learning, they offer meaningful learning experiences in which students learn and explore. Centers should not be just for fun experiences or time fillers, but for learning experiences based on targeted standards that are designed to meet the needs of a variety of learners. They are also great vehicles for offering students opportunities to use their various multiple intelligences. Figure 7.5 gives ample suggestions for centers and projects.

PROJECTS

What Are They?

A project is an in-depth study. Students explore a topic as investigators, researchers, and discoverers of knowledge. Projects can be varied and rich with opportunities for engaging learners and for deep understanding at a variety of levels of readiness, interests, or learning profiles. Projects are usually in a certain subject area dealing with a particular topic of study.

Projects can be assigned or chosen from a choice list or board. When deciding on a selection from the list, make sure each choice meets certain criteria:

- Has clear targeted standards
- Is age-appropriate so the students can do the assignment independently
- Teaches content being taught during the year
- Provides choices
- Fits an established timeline
- Is assessed by the established assessment tool

Structured Projects

In structured projects, the expectations and guidelines are structured and are shared with the students. Students work creatively to achieve success, given their understanding of concepts and the skills they have mastered. For example, in geometry, students are assigned the Building Project (build the tallest structure that will stand alone using the materials given). The project may be assigned to the whole class but responded to individually or in small groups.

Topic-Related Projects

These projects are typical, traditional school projects. Students choose a topic that interests and motivates them and produce a product that shows what has been learned or what is particularly significant to the learners. For example, students may choose a political figure, an issue, or a particular place or event associated with World War II that interests them.

Figure 7.5 Multiple Intelligences: Suggestions for Centers and Projects

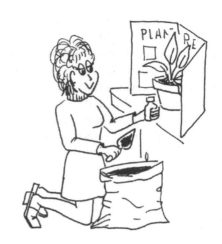

Verbal/Linguistic
Prepare a report.
Write a play or essay.
Create a poem or recitation.
Listen to an audiotape on . . .
Interview.
Label a diagram.
Give directions for . . .

Bodily/Kinesthetic
Create a role-play.
Construct a model or representation.
Develop a mime.
Create a tableau for . . .
Manipulate materials.
Work through a simulation.
Create actions for . . .

Musical/Rhythmic
Compose a rap song or rhyme.
Create a jingle to teach others.
Listen to musical selections about . . .
Write a poem.
Select music or songs for a particular
    purpose.

Naturalist
Discover or experiment.
Categorize materials or ideas.
Look for ideas from nature.
Adapt materials to a new use.
Connect ideas to nature.
Examine materials to make generalizations.

Visual/Spatial
Draw a picture.
Create a mural or display.
Illustrate an event.
Make a diagram.
Create a cartoon.
Paint or design a poster.
Design a graphic.
Use color to . . .

Interpersonal
Work with a partner or group.
Discuss and come to conclusions.
Solve a problem together.
Survey or interview others.
Dialogue about a topic.
Use cooperative groups.

Logical/Mathematical
Create a pattern.
Describe a sequence or process.
Develop a rationale.
Analyze a situation.
Critically assess . . .
Classify, rank, or compare . . .
Interpret evidence . . .
Timeline.

Intrapersonal
Think about and plan.
Write in a journal.
Review or visualize a way to do
    something.
Make a connection with past information or
    experiences.
Metacognitive moment.

Open-Ended Projects

These projects have minimal guidelines and few criteria and are loosely structured to encourage risk taking and creativity. These projects may be a challenge that causes students to draw on their knowledge and skills to produce a product that addresses the challenge. One middle school class looked at developing innovative products that would be useful to the elderly. The unit contained literacy skills as students developed questionnaires, surveys, and interviews to gather data from the elderly. They used the Internet to access information on trends and needs. They used principles of simple machines and other science and math skills. In a hands-on and creative component, they designed their inventions.

Why Do We Use Them?

Projects are used because they build on students' interest and satisfy curiosity. Students learn to plan their time and develop their research skills at various levels. Projects provide students with choices, ownership, and responsibility. They encourage independence and self-directed learning skills and allow students to work at complex and abstract levels that match their skill levels while managing time and materials. Projects are highly motivating and allow for in-depth work on interesting topics. Projects allow students to work at their own rates. However, they must be worth the academic time of the learner and be meaningful experiences, not just time fillers. Projects help learners interact with knowledge at a level higher than simple recall. They also help develop concepts more fully and enable students to construct their own understanding. Information learned in context with an emotional hook will be remembered longer if it is also a meaningful experience. Projects emphasize process as well as product and integrate many concepts, facts, and skills.

How Do We Use Them?

All projects need to be designed with the end in mind. That means the project is designed based on clear learning goals, standards, and content objectives. Projects should be age-appropriate and at the students' levels so the work is interesting and challenging without being overwhelming.

Teachers usually provide students with a suggestion list for projects. Design the list with a variety of intelligences targeted so that the learners can work on an area of strength for the presentation and format and because students' learning styles are diverse (see Figure 3.14 in Chapter 3, "Suggestions for Using the Eight Multiple Intelligences," and Figure 7.5, "Multiple Intelligences: Suggestions for Centers and Projects," earlier in this chapter). This allows learners to concentrate on information and spend time developing comprehension and a deeper understanding of the topic rather than always having to use verbal/linguistic models like essays, research papers, or oral presentations.

Procedure for Project Work

1. Choose a topic.

2. Develop a plan of action that includes a timeline, a distribution of duties if working in a group, and so on.

3. Implement the plan.

> Gather ideas
> List resources
> Decide on the format
> Refer to a rubric
> Conference
> Compile ideas
> Prepare a presentation

4. Display and present the project.

Evaluation: Self, Peer, Teacher, Significant Other

Students may be given the option to submit a contract for a project. This contract should meet the same criteria as the other suggested project assignments but would reflect the area of study chosen by the student. The student presents the contract to the teacher for approval. This is done best in a teacher-student conference so the learner can explain his or her thinking and ideas in detail. The teacher negotiates with the student until a reasonable contract is completed. Contracts may be proposed because the student has an interest in learning more about a particular area. This is important to learning because it satisfies the learner's personal learning needs. Students with a keen need and desire to learn will indeed learn more. They will be more committed and engaged and will invest more time and energy in the project.

Assessment

Rubrics are designed with clear criteria and indicators to establish expectations and the grading format. They include a detailed explanation of the requirements. Students should be clear up front about the criteria for success, and the rubric can guide them as they work on the project. The rubric informs the teacher, the student, and the parents about the requirements, guidelines, and expectations for the project from the beginning to the end (see Figure 7.6).

Students log and journal their timelines, findings, and procedures to show what they are learning, using, and processing. If working with others, they need to negotiate the workload and facilitate the project by using appropriate social skills. Students also need to reflect on the group's interactions as they work together. Teachers assign or students select the roles and duties for which they will be accountable.

Adjustable Projects

The teacher provides a range of resources matching the readiness levels of the students. The materials should be multilevel and age-appropriate. Adequate time must be spent on gathering and selecting the resources. Students select resources suitable for their projects and naturally choose materials that are appropriate to their readiness levels. Learners rarely choose materials that they can't read or understand.

Figure 7.6   Rubric for Project

Name _____

Project _____

Date _____

Self _____

Peer _____

Teacher _____

Accuracy of Information

2 _____ 3 _____ 4 _____ 5

Use of Visuals

2 _____ 3 _____ 4 _____ 5

Completion

2 _____ 3 _____ 4 _____ 5

Presentation

2 _____ 3 _____ 4 _____ 5

Team Member Involvement

2 _____ 3 _____ 4 _____ 5

Used Time Appropriately

2 _____ 3 _____ 4 _____ 5

Comments:

Thus projects are invariably adjusted as a matter of course because of the individuality of each student. A variety of multimedia and human resources can also be used for project work. The Internet and technology are valuable tools and should be considered for project work. They are intriguing and engaging for many learners and help develop the skills of accessing, gathering, and managing information.

Sample Projects

Integer Project

Math teacher Ellen Wilken (Granville, OH), who wanted her students to really understand integers, designed the following project choices.

Demonstrate knowledge of integer operations (+, −, =, x) by using one of the following projects:

1. Make an 8½ x 11 chart showing integer operation rules with examples.

2. Write a poem, newspaper article, or comic strip about integers.

3. Construct a three-dimensional art object, puzzle, or game that uses integer computation.

4. Write and perform a live or videotaped play.

5. Write and perform a song or jingle.

6. Interview someone outside the class about that person's understanding of integers. Record audio or video of the responses.

7. Write an autobiography about your understanding of integer computation and how it will help you in future situations.

8. Show evidence of integers in nature by use of photography, samples, or drawings.

She reported that students were highly engaged as they worked on their choices alone or with a partner. They had far greater understanding and ability to apply that understanding as a result of the project work.

Nutrition and Wellness Project

The following is an example of nutrition project choices that teacher Cindy Palur (Granville, OH) designed to consciously offer options in the area of multiple intelligences.

Action Project Ideas for Nutrition Class

If you are musical or rhythmic, you might like to

- Compose a song related to wellness
- Create a nutritional poem
- Make up a health-related rap song

If you like to write or talk, you might like to

- Write memos to be announced each morning to improve student wellness
- Create a nutritional commercial
- Write a report related to a wellness issue
- Create a nutritional brochure
- Read a nutritional or health-related book and make a report
- Interview a health professional and report your findings
- Keep a daily journal of your eating and exercise for a week and report on how they can be improved

If you like to dance or perform, you might like to

- Perform a play, dance, or skit depicting various elements of nutrition (eating disorders, coronary disease, etc.)
- Make a complete dinner for friends or family
- Create a routine or jazzercise dance to your favorite song and teach it to several friends
- Compose a poem or record audio or video of an element related to wellness

If you like to work with others, you might like to

- Volunteer at a food pantry or soup kitchen
- Volunteer to help a caterer
- Survey people who work in some aspect of nutrition and help them make positive changes to improve their levels of wellness; keep in touch as to their progress (e.g., set up an exercise or low-fat eating program)
- Organize an exercise or workout group and meet regularly
- Teach an elementary class an aspect of nutrition (e.g., "5 a Day")

If you like to use numbers or graphs or solve abstract problems, you might like to

- Collect data to make a graph to show the relationship of a health issue (e.g., Is there a relationship between students who eat five fruits and vegetables a day and normal weight?)
- Develop a board game
- Do a science experiment related to food (amount of fat, sugar, salt, acid base, etc.)
- Determine how many calories you need each day based on your size and level of activity and create a menu to reflect that number of calories
- Use a computer to create a nutritional or health brochure
- Compare and contrast various nutritional information (e.g., water vs. sports drinks)
- Do research related to food

If you like independent study and self-improvement, you might like to

- Keep a diary of your diet for a week and determine ways you can improve to meet the requirements of the Food Pyramid and Dietary Guidelines
- Plan family meals for a week and create a shopping list
- Set wellness goals and ways to accomplish them (e.g., gain weight, lose weight, exercise regularly) and keep track of your progress

- Attend a wellness conference, seminar, or workshop and report your findings

  If you like to draw or create, you might like to

- Draw a picture or poster depicting good nutrition for display in the cafeteria
- Create a new recipe and test it on friends or family
- Create an educational game around aspects of wellness or good nutrition
- Make a video showing good nutritional ideas
- Create new garnish ideas using food to entice young eaters to try new foods
- Draw an artistic wellness brochure

  If you are interested in nature and growing things, you might like to

- Grow your own food (e.g., tomatoes, cucumbers) and use it in a recipe
- Freeze, can, dry, or preserve food for later use (frozen corn, canned tomatoes, applesauce, jelly, frozen broccoli, dried apples, etc.)

Animal Project

Here is another example of project choices, created by a Chicago teacher, Jamie Downhower.

Your job is to teach the kindergarten and first-grade classes all about your animal. You are going to show them your trading card of your animal. You are also going to need to choose one of the items from the following list to create to put on display for our classroom zoo.

- Use a box to create a habitat that looks like the environment where your animal lives.
- Write a journal pretending that you are an animal expert who is observing your animal in the wild for a week. Be sure to write about what it does all day long.
- Pretend your animal is being taken to a country where no one has ever seen that kind of animal before. Write a newspaper article telling all about it; be sure to include information about what it eats, what it looks like, its size, its natural habitat, and so on.
- Write a story or a poem featuring your animal.
- Create a magazine advertisement encouraging people to donate money to help bring your animal to the Lincoln Park Zoo.
- Make a brochure educating people on all of the interesting facts about your animal.
- Make a life-sized picture of your animal, with lots of detail.
- Create a poster with important information about your animal.
- Draw a comic book featuring your animal.
- Design a map of the world, and show where your animal is originally from.
- Create a papier-mâché model of your animal.
- Make a pop-up book with your animal as the star.
- Create a food chain showing which animals eat your animal and which animals your animal eats.
- Write a letter to your state representatives telling them why your animal is important, and ask them to help take care of it.
- If you have a different idea, please ask me about it before you get started.

Migration Project

A variation of the animal project was used by Drew Tessler and Jamie Downhower (Chicago, IL) to create a Migration Project (see Figure 7.7).

Social Studies Project on the Bill of Rights

High school social studies teacher Keisha Gabriel (High Point, NC) used multiple intelligences when designing a unit about the Bill of Rights. She created a choice board for students to choose activities to demonstrate knowledge (see Figure 7.8).

Solar System Project

Figure 7.9 shows a choice board that Jamie Downhower (Chicago, IL) created for his class's unit on the Solar System.

CHOICE BOARDS

Choice boards give students multiple ways of processing information and rehearsing content and skills. Students may work alone or with one or more partners to accomplish the tasks they choose. Students may choose three in a row from a tic-tac-toe–style choice board and then make a free choice, or they may create their own tasks for a wild card. Choice boards can have multiple-choice lines, shapes, formats, and options (see Figures 7.10–7.12), and they may also be organized around multiple intelligences (see Figure 7.13).

PROBLEM-BASED LEARNING

What Is It?

Problem-based learning consists of providing students with ill-structured problems that are open-ended and challenging. Students use information and processes in real-world situations to solve the problems. Problem-based learning as a curriculum choice gives students the opportunity to work on problems in real-life scenarios. These problems are loosely structured and have no single right answer. They require investigation of options and application of the content and processes that students are studying and practicing. Students are required to form hypotheses and test their theories. They require that students use evidence from texts and other resources, make inferences, and support an opinion with an argument based on factual information.

Why Do It?

Howard Gardner (2004) defines *intelligence* as the ability to solve problems, handle crises, and produce something of value for one's culture. The ability to problem solve is an identified standard in most school districts and the Common Core State Standards. Students who learn only the facts may do well in a trivia game, but the ability to access information and use it practically and creatively (Sternberg, 1996) is

Figure 7.7 Sample Choice Board for Migration Project

Name _____ Date _____

Menu for Migration: Your job is to complete four activities this week—one from each box.

1.
A. What are the different things that we need to live? Draw a picture for each thing and write about why each is so important.
B. Create a Venn diagram (with two circles) to compare Ancient Peoples (Ancient Romans, Vikings, Earliest Americans, or other Ancient Peoples you have studied) to the modern lives that we have now.

2.
A. Find a partner and draw out the migration routes on the maps. Label these areas:
    Canada
    United States
    North America
    South America
    Mexico
    Atlantic, Pacific, and Arctic Oceans

3.
A. Imagine: A lot of your friends have gone across the Land Bridge.
Write a letter to your family persuading them to move to one of the areas below.
Let them know why you want to move.
What are your reasons for going across to a new continent?
Include a postcard of what life would be like from that place.
Choices:
    Arctic
    Mountains
    Seaside
    Tropical
    Plains
    Forests
    Around Lake Michigan
***Remember: Things won't look like they do now! This is over 10,000 years ago!

4.
A. You are in Chicago, and you are going to move to the desert during the summer. What would you need to live comfortably in the desert and to survive? Make a list and draw pictures of the items that you will need.
B. Write a short story where you are one of the first people on this continent. What is it like moving to a new place? What kinds of changes do you need to be ready for? Why choose one place over another? What hardships have you gone through to get to where you wanted to go?

Source: Created by Drew Tessler and Jamie Downhower, Chicago.

Figure 7.8 Bill of Rights Choice Board

Interpersonal Create a Bill of Rights for your school	Intrapersonal Journal: Explain how you use the First Amendment freedoms on a daily basis.	Visual/Spatial Video: *School House Rocks* Create a poster for each amendment with newspaper articles.
Bodily/Kinesthetic Role-Play: Constitutional Convention	**Wild Card!**	Naturalist Several scenarios of rights taken away. Student identifies which right and which amendment was in question.
Logical/Mathematical Timeline of events leading to the Constitution	Musical/Rhythmic Create a rap, poem, or song for the Bill of Rights	Verbal/Linguistic Mnemonic on First Amendment—RAPPS: Religion, Assembly, Petition, Press, Speech

a worthier goal because it is useful throughout life. Problem-based learning provides the brain with conditions that intrigue and engage. It allows for creative opportunities that provide learners with the chance to use their skills and capabilities in a variety of ways, use a range of resources, and balance their choices of learning with the teacher-directed objectives.

How Do We Do It?

Steps in Problem Solving

When students are solving problems, they must take the following steps:

- Clarify or identify the problem.
- Draw on background knowledge and experience.
- Begin with what you know.
- Plan your own approach.
- Work at your own pace.
- Use creative solutions.

Clarify the Problem

Through discussion and questioning, students identify the issues and discover the significant parts of the problem to address. A problem statement is then articulated.

Figure 7.9 Choice Board for Studying the Solar System

Science: Solar System: Study of the Planets

MUST DO:

Using the research sites bookmarked on our classroom computer, please choose one planet and use Kidspiration to prewrite an expository essay about what your planet looks like, how big it is, and what kind of gases are found on your planet. Please include lots of interesting facts you have learned from your research.

DO:

Use Kidspiration to create a word map. Include 12 facts: one about each planet and three other interesting facts about the solar system. Be sure to include pictures as well.

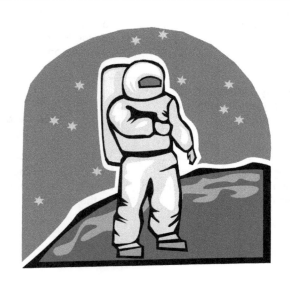

Write three specific questions about space that will later be e-mailed by the teacher to an astronaut at NASA.	Compare and contrast your planet with planet Earth. If your planet is Earth, choose any other planet to make your comparison.	Pretend you are an astronaut and write a diary entry to family on Earth about your day in space. Include what kind of experiments you did, what you ate, and where you slept.
Research the phases of the moon online and create a picture book with all of the phases and a one- or two-sentence summary of each phase. (Use the white paper by the project board to make your book.)	Your choice! Let's talk about it!	Pretend you are a travel agent and are creating a travel brochure for Chicago to attract visitors for all four seasons. Write about the kinds of weather that visitors can expect and draw lots of pictures to convince people to visit during each season.
Sketch your dream space shuttle. Please include as many details as possible and a paragraph describing your shuttle on the large paper near the project board.	Make a movie poster for a movie about space exploration. On the poster, include a drawing of the planets, sun, and moon.	Research constellations on the Internet or in one of our classroom books. Then create your own constellation using the star stickers on the project board. Write a story about how it was formed and why it is called by its name.

Source: Adapted from Jamie Downhower, Chicago Public Schools.

Figure 7.10 Sample Choice Board for Social Studies

Each student signs up to join a group to work on an area of interest. Make sure there are more "choice lines" than students so that everyone gets to select a favorite area.

Today's Country _____

Government	Geography	Beliefs and Rituals
1. _____	1. _____	1. _____
2. _____	2. _____	2. _____
3. _____	3. _____	3. _____
4. _____	4. _____	4. _____

People	Recreation	Occupations
1. _____	1. _____	1. _____
2. _____	2. _____	2. _____
3. _____	3. _____	3. _____
4. _____	4. _____	4. _____

Identify Resources

Students need to examine resources, including information and processes that they know from past experiences. A KND chart may be helpful for organizing this information (see Fogarty, 1998; Stepien, Gallagher, & Workman, 1993). The K stands for "What do you KNOW about this problem?" The N stands for "What do you NEED to solve this problem?" And the D stands for "What will you DO to get what you need?" Some teachers add a fourth element: P for PLAN. Students can often generate the first three columns but cannot get organized enough to proceed with their investigations. Planning is a step that many students need to think about. A plan may be modified as new ideas and information come up, but it helps students get started on their problem solving.

What do we Know? What do we Need to know? What can we Do? What is our Plan?

Figure 7.11 Sample Choice Wheel

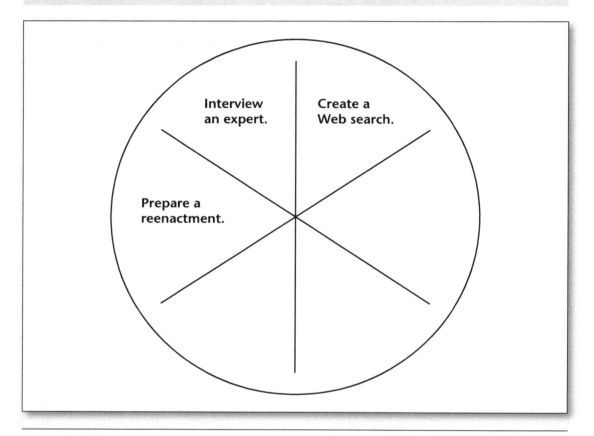

Accessing Information

Once students identify what they need to know, they can generate sources for that information or process. This gives them opportunities to use the Internet and other information-accessing systems.

Generating Hypotheses

After all information is uncovered and collected, students generate hypotheses for solutions.

Selecting and Rationalizing Solutions

A solution that students think best fits the problem is presented with backup rationale.

Sometimes, teachers ask students to take on an authentic role in the problem and to present to a real audience. One teacher asked students to work in groups as travel agents to design a trip to their state capital. They were to highlight the historical/ geographical features of the city/area and present their findings to parents with a

Figure 7.12 Choice Boards May Include Scrolls and Pyramids

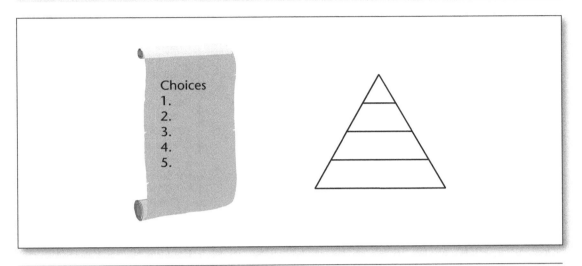

rationale as to why the class should visit the capital. This problem engaged learners in various ways. They were motivated to take the trip and find out what places would be interesting to visit and also to present that information to parents. The teacher had targeted the learning goals and then enticed the students to take ownership of the learning in a hands-on, practical way.

Secondary teacher Michael Bait gave his students the following instruction: "Construct an apparatus that can consistently project a steel ball to hit a target." He asked a group that needed a greater challenge to "hit a moving target."

A health education teacher presented the following to her students:

Group 1. As a sports nutritionist, create a menu plan for a week for a female athlete who weighs 130 pounds, is 5'5" tall, and plays on a soccer team.

Group 2. As a diet expert, create a menu plan for a week for a 15-year-old boy who wants to build muscle and put on weight before football season.

Group 3. During the next week, write down everything you eat and calculate the nutritional value as well as the caloric value. Use the computer program to help you.

She felt that these three groups of students would be challenged by these problems, so she provided a variety of contexts that would suit each one. Students in Group 3 were allowed the limited computer access available in the classroom because they needed that support to manage the calculations. The teacher's focus was on nutritional understanding and analysis, and she felt that the mathematical calculations would frustrate them and slow them down, thus losing their interest. Students were asked about their preferences before this assignment.

Posing problems with open-ended solutions is a great way to meet the learners where they are and engage them in accessing information and coming up with creative solutions. Problems are useful at any grade level and with almost any subject

Figure 7.13 Multiple Intelligences Choice Board

Verbal/Linguistic	Musical/Rhythmic	Visual/Spatial
Prepare a report Write a play or essay Give directions for . . . Create a poem or recitation Listen to a tape or view a video Retell in your own words Create a word web	Create a rap, song, or ballad Write a jingle Write a poem Select music to enhance a story or event Create rhymes that . . .	Create a mural, poster, or drawing Illustrate an event Draw a diagram Design a graphic organizer Use color to . . . Create a comic strip to show . . . Do a story board Create a collage with meaningful artifacts
Logical/Mathematical Create a pattern Describe a sequence or process Develop a rationale Analyze a situation Create a sequel Critically assess Classify, rank, or compare . . . Interpret evidence Design a game to show . . .	**Free Choice**	**Bodily/Kinesthetic** Create a role-play Construct a model or representation Develop a mime Create a tableau for . . . Manipulate materials to work through a simulation Create actions for . . .
Naturalist Discover or experiment Categorize materials or ideas Look for ideas from nature Adapt materials to a new use Connect ideas to nature Examine materials to make generalizations Label and classify Draw conclusions based on information Predict . . .	**Interpersonal** Work with a partner or group Discuss and come to conclusion Solve a problem together Survey or interview others Dialogue about a topic Use cooperative groups . . . to do a group project Project a character's point of view	**Intrapersonal** Think about and plan Write in a journal Keep track of . . . and comment on . . . Review or visualize a way Reflect on the character and express his or her feelings Image how it would feel if you . . .

matter. They are adjustable for different levels of readiness, complexity, and abstractness. As with projects, the students seek their levels of comfort and creativity and choose the "size that fits."

Inquiry, research, or independent study is another curricular model that engages students at their levels and interests. The inquiry model in Figure 7.14 is a simple flow chart that helps teachers take students through the process, beginning with an exploratory phase to define the topic, and build background experiences and knowledge. The next step is selecting a focus and posing a question that they wish to explore. They examine alternatives, consider and select the most appropriate one given their findings, and decide how to communicate their learning.

Figure 7.14   Flow Chart for a Basic Inquiry Model

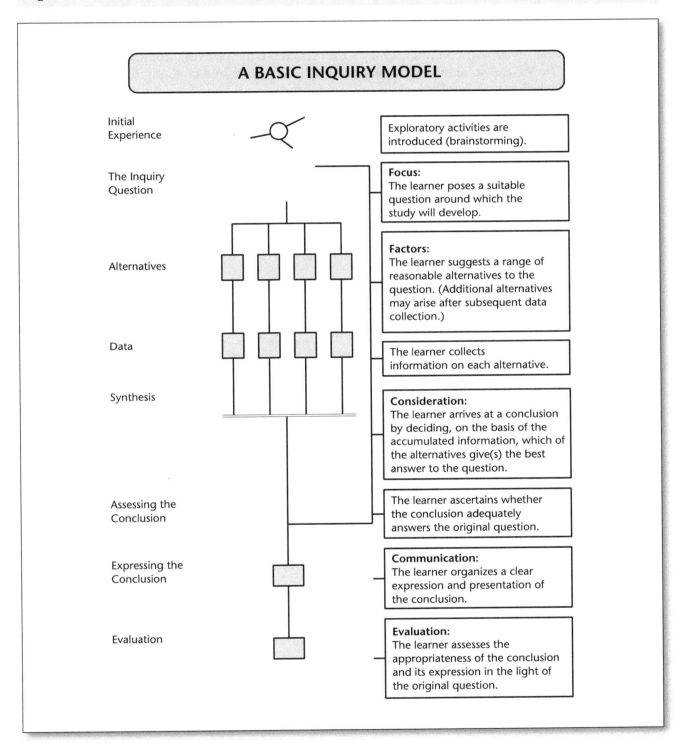

Source: From Ministry of Education, Ontario, *Research Study Skills: Curriculum Ideas for Teachers* (Toronto: Ministry of Education, 1979, p. 20).

ACADEMIC CONTRACTS

Contracts have often been used to allow students some flexibility and choice in their learning (Berte, 1975; Knowles, 1986; Robbins, Gregory, & Herndon, 2000; Tomlinson, 1998, 1999; Winebrenner, 1992). Contracts have the potential for students to develop "flow," the state in which they are totally engaged in a challenging and motivating task that matches their skills and preferences.

Academic contracts enable learners to do the following:

- Be clear about expectations
- Use their multiple intelligences
- Take ownership of their learning
- Learn to manage time and task

When teachers set up an academic contract, they consider the standards that will be targeted and the objectives in the subject content that will be embedded in the choices. Assessment tools, timelines, and clear expectations should be identified up front.

Figure 7.15 offers students eight choices for a culminating activity in a unit on World War II, plus a wild card for students to design an optional activity to be finished during the unit at their own pace. To use contracts, some class time would be given for conferencing with the teacher about choices and gathering resources. Students could also work on this project as a sponge activity whenever regular classwork was completed. After students select one of the options, they fill in the contract form (see Figure 7.16).

Some teachers use a double-duty log (see Figure 5.13 in Chapter 5) so students can keep track of time, process, and progress.

Another type of contract is one in which the teacher provides some core activities that all students will complete plus several options from which individual students can choose. An example is shown in Figure 7.17.

Sample Units That Use Contracts

Sample Unit 1: What Makes a Community?

Introduction: Over the next few weeks, we will be studying communities. You will be involved in many different activities that will help you understand why learning communities are established and how different people help keep a learning community working. Everyone in the class will complete some of the activities. You will be able to select other things to be completed on your own or with a group of your classmates.

Evaluation criteria:

- Thorough in-depth research
- All information is relevant
- Staying on task without reminders

Source: Used with permission from Sarward Baig and Linda Smeutek (Chicago, IL).

Figure 7.15 Choice Board for Study of World War II

1 Design four posters using your own drawings or pictures that depict the characteristics of life during World War II. Use captions to explain your visuals.	2 Develop an interview questionnaire; then interview at least four people who lived in this area during World War II. Describe at last five ways the war affected their lives.	3 Write and present a short one-act play that depicts life during World War II, either at home or overseas. Use support material from novels or historical references.
4 Read a book, such as *The Diary of Anne Frank,* and briefly describe four scenarios from the story showing how World War II changed the characters' lives.	5 Wild Card! Your choice. Please design an option and present it in writing by_____.	6 Produce a PowerPoint presentation using visuals, scripts, and sound to present life as one would have experienced it during World War II.
7 Listen to a variety of songs, musicals, and film soundtracks composed during World War II. Referring to the content of the songs, describe what the music conveys about what life was like during the war.	8 Collect a variety of pictures, newspaper articles, photographs, poems, and stories. Noting aspects of life during World War II, create a personal diary of how you would have felt growing up in that time.	9 Create a board game designed to increase understanding of what life was like during World War II.

Teacher Direction: Put a choice in each box. Use as many boxes as needed. There should be more lines on the total choice board than there are students in the classroom. This gives the last group a chance to have a selection.

Student Direction: Sign up for the one you choose.

Figure 7.16 Contract Form for Student to Fill In After Choosing an Activity

Name _____ Unit of Study _____

I agree to complete the following activity: _____

_____

I chose this option because _____

_____

_____

Please outline your plan: _____

_____

_____

_____

_____

_____

_____

_____

_____

_____

_____

_____

By the (date) _____

Signature _____

Figure 7.17   Contract Form In Which the Teacher Provides Some Core Activities

Author Study Contract

To help you improve your reading and writing, you will complete the core activities and may choose any optional activities that total at least 40 points.

Please fill in the contract and hand it in by _____.

Core Activities That Everyone Will Do: (Points)

1. I will select and begin a book by _____. (5)

2. I will create a "mind map" character sketch about a main character in my book (appearance, personality, friends/family, likes/dislikes). (10)

3. Each author uses language in interesting ways. Select 3 passages that you think are unique and explain in your own words their meaning and why you think the author expressed himself or herself in this way. (10)

Optional Selections:

4. I will write a dialogue that I could role-play about a situation or problem that I read (1 page). (10)

5. I will draw a story map or comic strip with captions outlining the plot. (10)

6. I will write a commercial, design a poster, or produce a brochure on the computer to advertise my book and/or the author. (5)

7. As a critic, I will write an article sharing my thoughts about the story, outlining what I thought was Plus, Minus, and Interesting (de Bono, 1987). This will be a full-page column. I will use the word-processing program on the computer. (10)

8. Design an option and discuss with the teacher. (5 or 10)

This will give me _____ points.

Signed by Student _____

Signed by Teacher _____

- Neatness
- Originality
- Working with others and helping the group
- Careful use of computer equipment

Directions: Read the list of activities below. When you decide on the activities you would like to complete on your own or with a group, please fill out the form, sign, and turn in the community Learning Contract Agreement at the end of this assignment.

Everyone in class will complete the following activities:

Done	Activity	Number of Points
	Using Inspiration software, create a mind map (concept map, many pictures) of your community.	10
	Find a problem in the community. How would you solve this problem?	5
	Make a book about "Where Do People Live?" Draw pictures and describe the different places you draw.	10
	Design a community model. Include the things you have learned about, such as libraries, banks, park buildings, museums, schools, hospitals, and police stations.	35
	Conduct an Internet search to find out about other communities and their workers. Listen to or read stories about their jobs.	10

Select from these optional activities so that your total project points will be at least 100.

Done	Activity	Points
	1. Create a travel brochure about your community. Your brochure should make people outside of your community want to come visit your community. How will you make your community seem special? What are some of the best things you can say about your community? Be sure to use pictures and words to make your brochure attractive and professional looking.	15
	2. Survey people (at least 10) in your community to find out their favorite places in the community. You might ask the following questions: What is your favorite restaurant? What is your favorite building? Who is your favorite veterinarian? First, decide how you will find out the information. Will you ask people yourself, or will you create a written survey to give them? How will you keep track of their responses? Finally, make a poster that shows your survey results. Show the favorite places in the community.	10
	3. What makes our community special? Draw pictures of people helping others, important community centers and places, and community events.	10

	4. Create a slideshow that clearly explains what a community is. The show should include the different types of community, community service workers, cultures, customs, and government. Include graphics (pictures, cartoons, maps, etc.).	15
	5. Complete a puzzle that shows a job within the community.	5
	6. What do you want to be? Draw a picture of the community helper you would like to be. Draw pictures of the helper's workplace and equipment.	10
	7. Design a building for a community, and write about why it is an important building for a community. Be sure to answer these questions: What is the name of the building? What makes it unique? How does it meet the needs of the people living in the community? What roles will people who work in the building play in the community?	10
	8. Use a computer program to draw a community map. Make sure to include a map key and cardinal directions.	10

What Makes a Community Contract? I, _____ agree to work on these activities to bring my total community unit points to at least 100. Here is a list of the extra activities I have chosen.

Extra Activities #1 and #2 Need Teacher Input	Points
1.	
2.	
3.	
4.	
5.	

I understand that my work will be evaluated based on the following criteria:

- Thorough in-depth research
- All information is relevant
- Staying on task without reminders
- Neatness
- Originality
- Working with others and helping the group finish a project
- Careful use of computer equipment

I understand that my contract work must be turned in by _____.

I will work on the contract activities that I select during class time unless I first discuss with my teacher doing something outside of class.

I agree to stay on task while working on my contract activities so that I do not distract others and so that I can put forth my best effort.

Student's Signature _____ Date _____

Teacher's Signature _____ Date _____

Sample Unit 2: Reading Workshop Contract

Week of_____

I agree to make just the right book selections and READ and READ so I can . . .
I will choose one from the following! Check off your choice.
I understand that I also need to continue my reading!

Assignment	*Done!*
Write a letter to _____	
Write a book recommendation	
Answer the question: Who is the trickiest villain: the big bad pig, Coyote, or the shark? Why? (Use support from the book to answer your question!)	

I agree to try my very best to complete all of my work. I will pay attention to directions and ask questions if things are unclear.

- Compare and contrast the Three Little Javelinas and the Three Hawaiian Pigs using a Venn diagram.
- Make up riddles for your vocabulary words. Have a partner try to figure them out!
- Collect shark facts and share them with the class.
- Write a letter to the shark giving him advice on a new disguise. Draw a picture of it.
- Write a paragraph describing a house that you would build if you were one of the pigs from the story. Answer the questions:

   What would it be made of?

   What would it look like?

   Where would it be?

   Draw a picture!

Signature _____ Date _____

Teachers need to ask certain questions as they plan and design a contract. Use the questions in Figure 7.18 to help plan contracts.

All these curriculum approaches allow for adjustments in the learning, offer variety guided by the standards, and engage learners with intriguing and thoughtful learning activities.

Source: Adapted from an idea from Ana Solis (Chicago, IL).

Figure 7.18 Questions Teachers Need to Ask Themselves as They Plan and Design Contracts

What are the standards, content, and skills that will be embedded in this contract? _____

_____

How long will the contract last? _____

What types of activities will support the standards and interest diverse learners? _____

_____

Brainstorm possibilities! _____

_____

What are the core activities that everyone will participate in? _____

_____

Should I design more than one contract considering the readiness of my students by examining the pre-assessment (simple-to-complex, concrete-to-abstract thinking)? _____

What weight should each task be assigned (points)? _____

Chapter 7
Reflections

1. In your professional learning communities, discuss and share the curriculum models you have used successfully in your classroom.

2. Share some personal tips and variations that helped you become successful using the following:

   Centers

   Projects

   Choice boards

   Problem-based learning

   Contracts

8

Putting It All Together in Your Differentiated Classroom

IN OUR QUEST TO FIND THE BEST FIT FOR OUR STUDENTS, WE NEED to recognize that change is a process, not an event (Fullan, 1991). This quest keeps us on a journey of continuous improvement.

Day-to-day planning takes time, especially when our planning involves the process of rethinking what we have accomplished in the one-size-fits-all classroom. We still "begin with the end in mind," focusing on the Common Core State Standards and expectations in the curriculum. We also adjust and redesign the learning activities, tailoring them to the needs and preferences of our unique learners in each classroom. We must use research-based, best practices when planning instruction. It is imperative for all of us to monitor our effectiveness in our efforts to maximize student learning.

Throughout this book, we present a treasure trove of ideas and strategies to fill your tool kits. Coming full circle in this chapter, we will revisit the lesson-planning template from Chapter 1 and the adjustable-assignments grid from Chapter 5. We apply the template and the grid (Figure 8.1) to plan differentiated lessons at various levels—early, elementary, middle, and high school. We use these organizational tools to differentiate content, interest, readiness, and multiple intelligences for the diverse learners—for those on the beginning level, approaching mastery or with a high degree of mastery. Differentiation does *not* mean always tiering every

Figure 8.1   The Six-Step Planning Model for Differentiated Learning: Template

Planning for Differentiated Learning	
1. STANDARDS: What should students know and be able to do?	Assessment tools for data collection: (logs, checklists, journals, agendas, observations, portfolios, rubrics, contracts)
Essential Questions:	
2. CONTENT: (concepts, vocabulary, facts) SKILLS:	
3. ACTIVATE: Focus Activity: Pre-assessment strategy Pre-assessment Prior knowledge & engaging the learners	• Quiz, test • Surveys • K-W-L • Journals • Arm gauge • Give me • Brainstorm • Concept formation • Thumb it
4. ACQUIRE: Total group or small groups	• Lecturette • Presentation • Demonstration • Jigsaw • Video • Field trip • Guest speaker • Text
5. Grouping Decisions: (TAPS, random, heterogeneous, homogeneous, interest, task, constructed) APPLY ADJUST	• Learning centers • Projects • Contracts • Compact/Enrichment • Problem based • Inquiry • Research • Independent study
6. ASSESS Diversity Honored (learning styles, multiple intelligences, personal interest, etc.)	• Quiz, test • Performance • Products • Presentation • Demonstration • Log, journal • Checklist • Portfolio • Rubric • Metacognition

lesson for three levels of complexity or challenge. It does mean finding interesting, engaging, and appropriate ways of honoring diversity to help students learn new concepts and skills. You are differentiating instruction each time you meet an individual's needs.

We believe it is important to start small but to think big, too. If you aim for one new, "gourmet" lesson each week, you'll have forty at the end of the year.

BODY SYSTEMS MIDDLE SCHOOL LESSON

The following CCSS will be targeted in the lesson on Skeletal and Muscular Systems, Figure 8.2:

ELA RST.6-8.1: Cite specific textual evidence to support analysis of science and technical texts.

ELA RST.6-8.3: Follow a precise multistep procedure when carrying out experiments, taking measurements, or performing technical tasks.

ELA RST.6-8.9: Compare and contrast the information gained from experiments, simulations, video or multimedia sources with knowledge gained from reading a text on the same topic.

ELA WHST.6-8.2: Write informative/explanatory texts, including the narration of historical events, scientific procedures/ experiments, or technical processes.

    b. Develop the topic with relevant, well-chosen facts, definitions, concrete details, quotations, or other information and examples.

    c. Use appropriate and varied transitions to create cohesion and clarify the relationships among ideas and concepts.

    d. Use precise language and domain-specific vocabulary to inform learners about or explain the topic.

Figure 8.2 Planning for Differentiated Learning for Middle School Science: Exploring the Functions of the Body's Skeletal and Muscular Systems

Planning for Differentiated Learning	
1. STANDARDS: What should students know and be able to do? Skeletal and muscular systems work together to carry out the life function of locomotion.	Assessment tools for data collection: (logs, checklists, journals, agendas, observations, portfolios, rubrics, contracts)
Essential Questions: What functions do skeletal and muscular systems provide? How do we better care for these systems?	
2. CONTENT: (concepts, vocabulary, facts) Muscles, skeleton, functions, ligaments, bones SKILLS: Visual representations / Cause and effect	
3. ACTIVATE: Focus Activity: Pre-assessment strategy Pre-assessment 3 Functions of skeletal/muscular system Prior knowledge 2 Questions you would like to ask & engaging the 1 Reason why this is good to know learners Label the parts of the skeletal & muscular systems	• Quiz, test • Surveys • K-W-L • Journals • Arm gauge • Give me • Brainstorm • Concept formation • Thumb it
4. ACQUIRE: Total group or small groups View video in groups of 3 with an advanced organizer. Small group discussion and fill in advance organizer as a summarizing and note-taking piece. Compare information from video with textbook reading working with a random partner.	• Lecturette • Presentation • Demonstration • Jigsaw • Video • Field trip • Guest speaker • Text
5. Grouping Decisions: (TAPS, random, heterogeneous, homogeneous, interest, task, constructed) APPLY ADJUST Students will group according to the choices they make from the choice board Students will work alone, in pairs or trios to complete two projects on the choice board. Students will present their projects from the choice board. Teacher and peers provide feedback with rubric.	• Learning centers • Projects • Contracts • Compact/Enrichment • Problem based • Inquiry • Research • Independent study
6. ASSESS Students will individually write a paper on the necessity and functions of the skeletal and muscular systems and their efforts to take care of these systems for healthy living. Test on parts and functions of the two systems. Diversity Honored (learning styles, multiple intelligences, personal interest, etc.)	• Quiz, test • Performance • Products • Presentation • Demonstration • Log, journal • Checklist • Portfolio • Rubric • Metacognition

HIGH SCHOOL AMERICAN HISTORY

In this lesson, the strategies for learning are differentiated. The teacher uses a quick informative pre-assessment to identify what the students know. Their interest is stimulated with a variety of audio, visual, and print materials and an ongoing discussion in cooperative small groups. Choice is provided with a Tic-Tac-Toe or Choice Board so students rehearse content and present their understandings in a variety of ways.

Remember, it is not necessary to differentiate each lesson with three levels of complexity or challenge. It is vital, however, to plan interesting, engaging, appropriate ways to learn new concepts and skills.

Targeted in this lesson dealing with American Immigration, Figure 8.3

ELA RH.11-12.1: Cite specific textual evidence to support analysis of primary and secondary sources, connecting insights gained from specific details to an understanding of the text as a whole.

ELA RH.11-12.2: Determine the central ideas or information of a primary or secondary source; provide an accurate summary that makes clear the relationships among the key details and ideas.

ELA RH.11-12.3: Evaluate various explanations for actions or events and determine which explanation best accords with textual evidence, acknowledging where the text leaves matters uncertain.

ELA RH.11-12.7: Integrate and evaluate multiple sources of information presented in diverse formats and media (e.g., visually, quantitatively, as well as in words) in order to address a question or solve a problem.

ELA WHST.11-12.9: Draw evidence from informational texts to support analysis, reflection, and research.

This lesson focuses on best practices of note-taking and summarizing using the four-corner organizer, so students can record the information about immigrant groups as a pre-assessment activity. Generating personal questions commits students to further investigation of the topic. Using an interest survey also helps students connect to the content in a personal way.

There are a variety of resources to facilitate investigation of immigrant groups. TAPS is used throughout the learning experience. The total group completes an interest survey. Learners identify personal interests independently. Students work in pairs and small groups at various different times. Students have multiple rehearsals using a variety of instructional strategies. Learning styles are respected: auditory, visual, tactile. Always remember that one size doesn't fit all!

Figure 8.4 offers reflection questions for teachers to ask as they move toward differentiated learning for their students.

Figure 8.3   Planning for Differentiated Learning for High School Social Studies: Examining the Impact of European Immigration on American Culture

Planning for Differentiated Learning	
1. STANDARDS: What should students know and be able to do? Examine the influx of European immigrants and their contributions to American society.	Assessment tools for data collection: (logs, checklists, journals, agendas, observations, portfolios, rubrics, contracts)
Essential Questions: How has the ethnicity of immigrants in the early 21st century influenced and affected our lives in the United States?	
2. CONTENT: (concepts, vocabulary, facts) Immigration, culture, emigration, relocation, ethnicity, employment, religion	SKILLS: Compare and contrast. Research and data collection. Visual representation.
3. ACTIVATE: Focus Activity: Pre-assessment strategy Pre-assessment Prior knowledge & engaging the learners Students create a four-corner organizer to fill in what they know about immigration at the beginning of the 21st century. Each student will generate a personal question. Guest speaker: immigrant grandparent.	• Quiz, test • Surveys • K-W-L • Journals • Arm gauge • Give me • Brainstorm • Concept formation • Thumb it
4. ACQUIRE: Total group or small groups From an interest survey, students identify which groups of immigrants they would like to investigate more thoroughly. Students will use the Internet, text, resource center, and community resources to gather information on a W5 chart.	• Lecturette • Presentation • Demonstration • Jigsaw • Video • Field trip • Guest speaker • Text
5. Grouping Decisions: (TAPS, random, heterogeneous, homogeneous, interest, task, constructed) APPLY ADJUST Students in small groups will present their findings to the total class. Each student will partner with another student who investigated a different ethnicity of immigrants using a cross-classification matrix. Students will regroup until the entire chart is filled in and all students have discussed all immigrant groups.	• Learning centers • Projects • Contracts • Compact/Enrichment • Problem based • Inquiry • Research • Independent study
6. ASSESS Students will create a "mindmap" in small groups to symbolize the contributions of immigrants to the American culture. Test on immigration in the early 21st century and the impact of the different ethnic groups. Diversity Honored (learning styles, multiple intelligences, personal interest, etc.)	• Quiz, test • Performance • Products • Presentation • Demonstration • Log, journal • Checklist • Portfolio • Rubric • Metacognition

Figure 8.4 Checklist of Questions for Teachers Planning Differentiated Learning for Their Students

B uilding Safe Environments
- Do students feel safe to risk and experiment with ideas?
- Do students feel included in the class and supported by others?
- Are tasks challenging enough without undo or "dis" stress?
- Is there an emotional "hook" for the learners?
- Are there novel, unique, and engaging activities to capture and sustain attention?
- Are "unique brains" honored and provided for? (learning styles & multiple intelligences)

R ecognizing and Honoring Diversity
- Does the learning experience appeal to the learners' varied and multiple intelligences and learning styles?
- May the students work collaboratively and independently?
- May they "show what they know" in a variety of ways?
- Does the cultural background of the learners influence instruction?

A ssessment
- Are pre-assessments given to determine readiness?
- Is there enough time to explore, understand, and transfer the learning to long-term memory (grow dendrites)? Is there time to accomplish mastery?
- Do they have opportunities for ongoing, "just in time" feedback?
- Do they have time to revisit ideas and concepts to connect or extend them?
- Is metacognitive time built into the learning process?
- Do students use logs and journals for reflection and goal setting?

I nstructional Strategies
- Are the expectations clearly stated and understood by the learner?
- Will the learning be relevant and useful to the learner?
- Does the learning build on past experience or create a new experience?
- Does the learning relate to their real world?
- Are strategies developmentally appropriate and hands on?
- Are the strategies varied to engage and sustain attention?
- Are there opportunities for projects, creativity, problems, and challenges?

N umerous Curriculum Approaches
- Do students work alone, in pairs, and in small groups?
- Do students work in learning centers based on interest, need, or choice?
- Are some activities adjusted to provide appropriate levels of challenge?
- Is pretesting used to allow for compacting/enrichment?
- Are problems, inquires, and contracts considered?

Schools are better right now than they have ever been. Teachers are assessing before, during, and after the learning more than ever. Many are interpreting the data and using the data to plan. More effective lessons are being taught. But even though there has been growth and progress in bringing quality to the differentiated classrooms, there is still room for improvement. Here are some ways to improve and continue to grow:

- Use lecturettes and improve in chunking information that fits while integrating curriculum.
- Continue to learn to incorporate new and stimulating instructional tools to teach the Common Core State Standards.
- Build a learning culture in which learners can take risks, feel safe, and know that you believe in them.
- Build in stimulating assignments to increase student engagement.
- Learn more about individual students and their needs in order to build a learning profile.
- Stop wasting time. It is a waste of your time to teach unnecessary lessons that do not address the Common Core State Standards.
- Allow students to peer and self-assess in order to get instant feedback so that they can learn about their errors and validate the parts that are right. This also will free up time for you to concentrate on students who need more direct teacher attention.
- Remember, one size doesn't fit all!

Bibliography

Anderson, L., & Krathwohl, D. (Eds.). (2001). *A taxonomy for learning, teaching, and assessing: A revision of Bloom's taxonomy of educational objectives.* New York, NY: Addison-Wesley Longman.

Aronson, E. (1978). *The jigsaw classroom.* Beverly Hills, CA: Sage.

Baumeister, R. F., & Vohs, K. D. (2006). *Handbook of self-regulation: Research, theory and applications* (2nd ed.). New York, NY: Guilford Press.

Bellanca, J., & Fogarty, R. (1991). *Blueprints for thinking in the cooperative classroom.* Thousand Oaks, CA: Corwin.

Bennett, B., Rolheiser-Bennett, C., & Stevahn, L. (1991). *Cooperative learning: Where heart meets mind.* Toronto, Ontario, Canada: Educational Connections.

Berte, N. (1975). *Individualizing education by learning contracts.* San Francisco, CA: Jossey-Bass.

Black, P., Harrison, C., Lee, C., Marshall, B., & Wiliam, D. (2004). Working inside the black box: Assessment for learning in the classroom. *Phi Delta Kappan, 86*(1), 8–21.

Black, P., & Wiliam, D. (2009). Developing the theory of formative assessment. *Educational Assessment, Evaluation, and Accountability, 21,* 5–31.

Bloom, B. S., et al. (1956). *Taxonomy of educational objectives. Handbook 1: Cognitive domain.* New York, NY: David McKay.

Brain, M. (2000). *How laughter works.* Retrieved from http://health.howstuffworks.com/mental-health/human-nature/other-emotions/laughter.htm

Brooks, J., & Brooks, M. (1993). *In search of understanding: The case for constructivist classrooms.* Alexandria, VA: Association for Supervision and Curriculum Development.

Brooks, R., & Goldstein, S. (2008). The mindset of teachers capable of fostering resilience in students. *Canadian Journal of School Psychology, 23,* 114–126.

Burke, K. (1993). *The mindful school: How to assess authentic learning.* Thousand Oaks, CA: Corwin.

Burke, K. (2009). *How to assess authentic learning* (5th ed.). Thousand Oaks, CA: Corwin.

Burke, K., Fogarty, R., & Belgrad, S. (1994). *The portfolio connection.* Thousand Oaks, CA: Corwin.

Caine, G., Caine, R. N., & Crowell, S. (1994). *Mindshifts: A brain-based process for restructuring schools and renewing education.* Tucson, AZ: Zephyr.

Caine, R. N., & Caine, G. (1991). *Making connections: Teaching and the human brain.* Alexandria, VA: Association for Supervision and Curriculum Development.

Caine, R. N., & Caine, G. (1994). *Making connections: Teaching and the human brain.* Reading, MA: Addison-Wesley.

Caine, R. N., & Caine, G. (1997). *Education on the edge of possibility.* Alexandria, VA: Association for Supervision and Curriculum Development.

Campbell, D. (1998). *The Mozart effect.* New York, NY: Avon.

Cantelon, T. (1991a). *The first 4 weeks of cooperative learning.* Portland, OR: Prestige.

Cantelon, T. (1991b). *Structuring the classroom successfully for cooperative team learning.* Portland, OR: Prestige.

Cardoso, S. H. (2000). Our ancient laughing brain. *Cerebrum: The Dana Forum on Brain Science, 2*(4), 15–30.

Chapman, C. (1993). *If the shoe fits: How to develop multiple intelligences in the classroom.* Thousand Oaks, CA: Corwin.

Chapman, C., & King, R. (2000). *Test success in the brain-compatible classroom.* Tucson, AZ: Zephyr Press.

Chapman, C., & King, R. (2005). *Differentiated assessment strategies: One tool doesn't fit all.* Thousand Oaks, CA: Corwin.

Chapman, C., & King, R. (2007a). *Differentiated reading and writing strategies for elementary classrooms* (Multimedia kit). Thousand Oaks, CA: Corwin.

Chapman, C., & King, R. (2007b). *Differentiated reading and writing strategies for secondary classrooms* (Multimedia kit). Thousand Oaks, CA: Corwin.

Chapman, C., & King, R. (2008). *Differentiated instructional management: Work smarter, not harder.* Thousand Oaks, CA: Corwin.

Chapman, C., & King, R. (2009a). *Differentiated instructional strategies for reading in the content areas* (2nd ed.). Thousand Oaks, CA: Corwin.

Chapman, C., & King, R. (2009b). *Differentiated instructional strategies for writing in the content areas* (2nd ed.). Thousand Oaks, CA: Corwin.

Chapman, C., & Vagle, N. (2011). *Motivating students: 25 strategies to light the fire of engagement.* Bloomington, IN: Solution Tree Press.

Cherniss, C., & Goleman, D. (2001). *The emotionally intelligent workplace: How to select for, measure, and improve emotional intelligence in individuals, groups, and organizations.* San Francisco, CA. Jossey-Bass.

Clarke, J., Wideman, R., & Eadie, S. (1990). *Together we learn.* Scarborough, Ontario, Canada: Prentice Hall.

Costa, A. (1995). *Outsmarting IQ: The emerging science of learnable intelligence.* Old Tappan, NJ: Free Press.

Cowan, G., & Cowan, E. (1980). *Writing.* New York, NY: John Wiley & Sons.

Csikszentmihalyi, M. (1990). *Flow: The psychology of optimal experience.* New York, NY: HarperCollins.

Damasio, A. R. (1994). *Descartes' error.* New York, NY: Putnam.

Darling-Hammond, L., Barron, B., Pearson, P.D., Schoenfeld, A. H., Stage, E. K., Zimmerman, T. D., . . . & Tilson, J. L. (2008). *Powerful learning: What we know about teaching for understanding.* San Francisco, CA: John Wiley & Sons.

de Bono, E. (1987). *CoRT thinking program.* Elmsford, NY: Pergamon.

Dean, C. B., Hubbell, E. R., Pitler, H., & Stone, B. J. (2012). *Classroom instruction that works: Research-based strategies for increasing student achievement* (2nd ed.). Alexandria, VA: Association for Supervision and Curriculum Development.

DePorter, B., Reardon, M., & Singer-Nourie, S. (1998). *Quantum teaching: Orchestrating student success.* Boston, MA: Allyn & Bacon.

Diamond, M. (2001). Response of the brain to enrichment. *Annals of the Brazilian Academy of Sciences, 73,* 211–220.

Donavan, S., & Bransford, J. D. (2005). *How students learn history, mathematics, and science in the classroom.* Washington, DC: National Academies Press.

Doyle, M., & Strauss, D. (1976). *How to make meetings work.* New York, NY: Playboy.

Driscoll, M. E. (1994, April). *School community and teacher's work in urban settings: Identifying challenges to community in the school organization.* Paper presented at the annual meeting of the American Educational Research Association, New Orleans, LA.

Dunn, K., & Dunn, R. (1992). *Bringing out the giftedness in your child.* New York, NY: John Wiley & Sons.

Dunn, R., & Dunn, K. (1987). Dispelling outmoded beliefs about student learning. *Educational Leadership, 44*(6), 55–61.

Dweck, C. S. (2006). *Mindset: The new psychology of success.* New York, NY: Random House.

Earl, L. (2003). *Assessment as learning: Using classroom assessment to maximize student learning.* Thousand Oaks, CA: Corwin.

Ekwall, E. E., & Shanker, J. L. (1988). *Diagnosis and remediation of the disabled reader* (3rd ed.). Boston, MA: Allyn & Bacon.

Fogarty, R. (1998). *Problem-based learning and other curricular models for the multiple intelligences classroom.* Thousand Oaks, CA: Corwin.

Fogarty, R., & Stoehr, J. (1995). *Integrating curricula with multiple intelligences: Teams, themes, and threads.* Thousand Oaks, CA: Corwin.

Frey, N., Fisher, D., & Everlove, S. (2009). *Productive group work: How to engage students, build teamwork, and promote understanding.* Alexandria, VA: Association for Supervision and Curriculum Development.

Fullan, M. (with Steigelbauer, S.). (1991). *The new meaning of educational change.* New York, NY: Teachers College Press.

Gardner, H. (2004). *Frames of mind: The theory of multiple intelligences* (20th anniv. ed.). New York, NY: Basic Books.

Gardner, H. (2006). *Multiple intelligences: New horizons in theory and practice.* New York, NY: Basic Books.

Gay, G. (2000). *Culturally responsive teaching: Theory, research, and practice.* New York, NY: Teachers College Press.

Geake, J. G. (2009). *The brain at school: Educational neuroscience in the classroom.* New York, NY: McGraw-Hill.

Gibbs, J. (1995). *Tribes: A new way of learning and being together.* Santa Rosa, CA: Center Source.

Glasser, W. (1990). *The quality school.* New York, NY: Harper & Row.

Glasser, W. (1998). *Choice theory in the classroom.* New York, NY: HarperCollins.

Goleman, D. (1995). *Emotional intelligence.* New York, NY: Bantam.

Goleman, D. (1998). *Working with emotional intelligence.* New York, NY: Bantam.

Goleman, D. (2006). Teaching to student strengths: The socially intelligent leader. *Educational Leadership, 64*(1), 76–81.

Goodwin, B., Lefkowits, L., Woempner, C., & Hubbell, E. (2012). *The future of schooling: Educating America in 2020.* Bloomington, IN: Solution Tree.

Green, E. J., Greenough, W. T., & Schlumpf, B. E. (1983). Effects of complex or isolated environments on cortical dendrites of middle-aged rats. *Brain Research, 264,* 233–240.

Gregorc, A. (1982). *Inside styles: Beyond the basics.* Columbia, CT: Gregorc Associates.

Gregory, G. H. (2005). *Differentiating instruction with style.* Thousand Oaks, CA: Corwin.

Gregory, G. H. (2008). *Differentiated instructional strategies in practice.* Thousand Oaks, CA: Corwin.

Gregory, G. H., & Kaufeldt, M. (2012). *Think big, start small: How to differentiate instruction in a brain-friendly classroom.* Bloomington, IN. Solution Tree Press.

Gregory, G. H., & Kuzmich, L. (2004). *Data-driven differentiation in the standards-based classroom.* Thousand Oaks, CA: Corwin.

Gregory, G. H., & Kuzmich, L. (2005a). *Differentiated literacy strategies for student growth and achievement in grades K–6.* Thousand Oaks, CA: Corwin.

Gregory, G. H., & Kuzmich, L. (2005b). *Differentiated literacy strategies for student growth and achievement in grades 7–12.* Thousand Oaks, CA: Corwin.

Gregory, G. H., & Kuzmich, L. (2007). *Teacher teams that get results: 61 group process skills and strategies.* Thousand Oaks, CA: Corwin.

Gregory, G. H., & Kuzmich, L. (2008). *Student teams that get results: 61 group process skills and strategies.* Thousand Oaks, CA: Corwin.

Gregory, G. H., & Parry, T. S. (2006). *Designing brain-compatible learning* (3rd ed.). Thousand Oaks, CA: Corwin.

Gurian, M., Henley, P., & Trueman, T. (2001). *Boys and girls learn differently: A guide for teachers and parents.* San Francisco, CA: Jossey-Bass.

Gurian, M., & Stevens, K. (2005). *The minds of boys: Saving our sons from falling behind in school and life.* San Francisco, CA: Jossey-Bass.

Hallowell, E. M. (2011). *Shine: Using brain science to get the best from your people.* Boston, MA: Harvard Business School.

Hanson, J. R., & Silver, H. F. (1978). *Learning styles and strategies.* Moorestown, NJ: Hanson Silver Strong.

Hargreaves, S., & Fullan, M. (1998). *What's worth fighting for out there?* New York, NY: Teachers College Press.

Harmin, M. (1994). *Inspiring active learning.* Alexandria, VA: Association for Supervision and Curriculum Development.

Hart, L. A. (1998). *Human brain and human learning.* Kent, WA: Books for Educators.

Healy, J. (1992). *Endangered minds: Why our children don't think.* New York, NY: Simon & Schuster.

Healy, J. (2010). *Different learners: Identifying, preventing, and treating your child's learning problems.* New York, NY: Simon & Schuster.

Hill, S., & Hancock, J. (1993). *Reading and writing communities.* Armadale, Australia: Eleanor Curtin.

Hunter, R. (2004). *Madeline Hunter's mastery teaching: Increasing instructional effectiveness in elementary and secondary schools* (Rev. ed.). Thousand Oaks, CA: Corwin.

Hyerle, D. (2009). *Visual tools for transforming information into knowledge.* Thousand Oaks, CA: Corwin.

Immordino-Yang, M. H., & Damasio, A. (2007). We feel, therefore we learn: The relevance of affective and social neuroscience to education. *Mind, Brain, and Education, 1*(1), 3–10.

Jensen, E. (1996). *Completing the puzzle: The brain-based approach.* Del Mar, CA: Turning Points.

Jensen, E. (1998a). *Introduction to brain-compatible learning.* Thousand Oaks, CA: Corwin.

Jensen, E. (1998b). *Teaching with the brain in mind.* Alexandria, VA: Association for Supervision and Curriculum Development.

Johnson, D. W., & Johnson, F. P. (2009). *Joining together* (10th ed.). Upper Saddle River, NJ: Pearson.

Johnson, D. W., Johnson, R. T., & Holubec, E. J. (1998). *Cooperation in the classroom.* Edina, MN: Interaction Book.

Kagan, S. (1992). *Cooperative learning.* San Clemente, CA: Kagan.

Knowles, M. (1986). *Using learning contracts.* San Francisco, CA: Jossey-Bass.

Kolb, D. (1984). *Experiental learning: Experience as the source of learning and development.* Englewood Cliffs, NJ: Prentice Hall.

Kotulak, R. (1996). *Inside the brain: Revolutionary discoveries of how the mind works.* Kansas City, MO: Andrews & McMeely.

LeDoux, J. (1996). *The emotional brain.* New York, NY: Simon & Schuster.

Lou, Y., Alorami, P. C., Spence, J. C., Paulsen, C., Chambers, B., & d'Apollonio, S. (1996). Within-class grouping: A meta-analysis. *Review of Educational Research, 66*, 423–458.

Lyman, F., & McTighe, J. (1988). Cueing thinking in the classroom: The promise of theory-embedded tools. *Educational Leadership, 5*(7), 18–24.

Marzano, R. J. (1992). *A different kind of classroom teaching with dimensions of learning.* Alexandria, VA: Association for Supervision and Curriculum Development.

Marzano, R. J. (2007). *The art and science of teaching: A comprehensive framework for effective instruction.* Alexandria, VA: Association for Supervision and Curriculum Development.

Marzano, R. J., & Brown, J. L. (2009). *A handbook for the art and science of teaching.* Alexandria, VA: Association for Supervision and Curriculum Development.

Marzano, R. J., Pickering, D. J., & Pollack, J. E. (2001). *Classroom instruction that works.* Alexandria, VA: Association for Supervision and Curriculum Development.

Maslow, A. (1954). *Motivation and personality.* New York, NY: Harper & Row.

Maslow, A. (1968). *Toward a psychology of being.* New York, NY: Van Nostrand Reinhold.

McCarthy, B. (1990). Using the 4MAT system to bring learning styles to schools. *Educational Leadership, 48*(2), 31–37.

McCarthy, B., & McCarthy, D. (2006). *Teaching around the 4MAT cycle: Designing instruction for diverse learners with diverse learning styles.* Thousand Oaks, CA: Corwin.

McMillan, J. H. (Ed.). (2007). *Formative classroom assessment: Theory into practice.* New York, NY: Teachers College Press.

McTighe, J. (1990). *Better thinking and learning.* [Workshop handout]. Baltimore: Maryland State Department of Education.

Miller, G. (1956). The magical number seven, plus or minus two: Some limits on our capacity for processing information. *Psychological Review, 63,* 81–97.

Pianta, R. C., Hitz, R., & West, B. (2010). *Increasing the application of developmental sciences knowledge in educator preparation: Policy and practice issues.* Washington, DC: National Council for Accreditation of Teacher Education. Retrieved from http://www.ncate.org/LinkClick.aspx?fileticket=OGdzx714RiQ%3D&tabid=706

National Institute of Child Health and Human Development. (2004). *Teaching children to read: An evidence-based assessment of the scientific research literature on reading and its implications for reading instruction.* Washington, DC: Government Printing Office.

Ogle, D. (1986). K-W-L: A teaching model that develops active reading of expository text. *Reading Teacher, 39,* 564–574.

O'Keefe, J., & Nadel, L. (1978). *The hippocampus as a cognitive map.* Oxford, UK: Clarendon.

Ornstein, R., & Thompson, R. (1984). *The amazing brain.* Boston, MA: Houghton Mifflin.

Panksepp, J. (1998). *Affective neuroscience: The foundations of human and animal emotions.* New York, NY: Oxford University Press.

Pascal-Leon, J. (1980). Compounds, confounds, and models in developmental information processing: A reply to Trabasso and Foellinger. *Journal of Experimental Child Psychology, 1,* 18–40.

Paulson, F. L., Paulson, P. R., & Meyer, C. A. (1991). What makes a portfolio a portfolio? *Educational Leadership, 48*(5), 60–63.

Pert, C. B. (1998). *Molecules of emotion.* New York, NY: Scribner.

Peterson, L. R., & Peterson, M. J. (1959). Short-term retention of individual verbal items. *Journal of Experimental Psychology, 58,* 193–198.

Pinker, S. (1998). *How the mind works.* New York, NY: Norton.

Popham, W. J. (2006). Phony formative assessment: Buyer beware. *Educational Leadership, 64*(3), 86–87.

Prensky, M. (2010). *Teaching digital natives: Partnering for real learning.* Thousand Oaks, CA: Corwin.

Prestidge, L. K., & Williams Glaser, C. H. (2000). Authentic assessment: Employing appropriate tools for evaluating students' work in 21st-century classrooms. *Intervention in School & Clinic, 35,* 178–182.

Ratey, J. J. (2008). *Spark: The revolutionary new science of exercise and the brain.* New York, NY: Little, Brown.

Reeves, D. (2000). Standards are not enough: Essential transformations for school success. *NASSP Bulletin, 84,* 5–19.

Reis, S., & Renzulli, J. (1992). Using curriculum compacting to challenge the above average. *Educational Leadership, 50*(2), 51–57.

Restak, R. (1993). *The brain has a mind of its own.* New York, NY: Harmony.

Robbins, P., Gregory, G., & Herndon, L. (2000). *Thinking inside the block schedule.* Thousand Oaks, CA: Corwin.

Rolheiser, C., Bower, B., & Stevahn, L. (2000). *The portfolio organizer.* Alexandra, VA: Association for Supervision and Curriculum Development.

Rowe, M. B. (1988, Spring). Wait time: Slowing down may be a way of speeding up. *Educator,* p. 43.

Rozman, D. (1998, March). Speech given at the Symposium on the Brain. Berkeley: University of California, Berkeley.

Sapolsky, R. M. (1998). *Why zebras don't get ulcers.* New York, NY: Freeman.

Sax, L. (2005). *Why gender matters.* New York, NY: Doubleday.

Shanker, S., & Downer, R. (2012). Enhancing the potential in children (EPIC). In L. Miller & D. Hevey (Eds.), *Policy issues in the early years* (pp. 61–76). London, UK: Sage.

Shepard, L. (2006, June). *Integrating assessment with instruction: What will it take to make it work.* Panel presentation at the National Large-Scale Assessment Conference, San Francisco, CA.

Silver, H. F., & Perini, M. (2010). The 8 C's of engagement: How learning styles and instructional design increase student commitment to learning. In R. Marzano (Ed.), *On excellence in teaching* (pp. 319–344). Bloomington, IN: Solution Tree Press.

Silver, H. F., Strong, R. W., & Perini, M. J. (2000). *So each may learn: Integrating learning styles and multiple intelligences.* Alexandria, VA: Association for Supervision and Curriculum Development.

Slavin, R. E. (1994). *Cooperative learning: Theory, research, and practice.* Boston, MA: Allyn & Bacon.

Smith, F. (1986). *Insult to intelligence.* New York, NY: Arbor House.

Sousa, D. A. (2006). *How the brain learns* (3rd ed.). Thousand Oaks, CA: Corwin.

Sousa, D. A. (Ed.). (2010). *Mind, brain, and education: Neuroscience implications for the classroom.* Bloomington, IN: Solution Tree Press.

Sousa, D. A. (2011). *What principals need to know about the basics of creating brain-compatible classrooms.* Bloomington, IN: Solution Tree Press.

Sousa, D. A., & Tomlinson, C. A. (2010). *Differentiation and the brain: How neuroscience supports the learner-friendly classroom.* Bloomington, IN: Solution Tree Press.

Sprenger, M. (1998). *Learning and memory: The brain in action.* Alexandria, VA: Association for Supervision and Curriculum Development.

Stepien, W., Gallagher, S., & Workman, D. (1993). Problem-based learning for traditional and interdisciplinary classrooms. *Journal for Gifted Education, 16,* 338–357.

Sternberg, R. (1996). *Successful intelligence: How practical and creative intelligence determine success in life.* New York, NY: Simon & Schuster.

Stiggins, R. (1993). *Student-centered classroom assessment.* Englewood Cliffs, NJ: Prentice Hall.

Stiggins, R. J. (2001). *Student-involved classroom assessment* (3rd ed.). Upper Saddle River, NJ: Merrill Prentice Hall.

Stiggins, R. J., Arter, J, Chappuis, J., & Chappuis, S. (2006). *Classroom assessment for student learning: Doing it right: Using it well.* Princeton, NJ: Merrill Prentice Hall.

Sylwester, R. (1995). *A celebration of neurons: An educator's guide to the brain.* Alexandria, VA: Association for Supervision and Curriculum Development.

Tapscott, D. (2009). *Grown up digital: How the net generation is changing your world.* New York, NY: McGraw-Hill.

Tilly, D. (2009). Questions and answers on response to intervention. *Journal of Special Education Leadership, 50*(4), 7, 12.

Tomlinson, C. A. (1998). *Differentiating instruction: Facilitator's guide.* Alexandria, VA: Association for Supervision and Curriculum Development.

Tomlinson, C. A. (1999). *The differentiated classroom: Responding to the needs of all learners.* Alexandria, VA: Association for Supervision and Curriculum Development.

Tomlinson, C. A. (2001). *How to differentiate instruction in mixed-ability classrooms* (2nd ed.). Alexandria, VA: Association for Supervision and Curriculum Development.

Vygotsky, L. S. (1978). *Mind in society: The development of higher psychological processes.* Cambridge, MA: Harvard University Press.

Vygotsky, L. S. (1993). *The collected works of L. S. Vygotsky. Volume 2: The fundamentals of defectology* (J. E. Knox & C. B. Stevens, Trans., R. W. Rieber & A. S. Carton, Eds.). New York, NY: Plenum Press.

Wiggins, G., & McTighe, J. (1998). *Understanding by design.* Alexandria, VA: Association for Supervision and Curriculum Development.

Willis, J. (2010). Want children to "pay attention"? Make their brains curious! *Psychology Today.* Retrieved from http://www.psychologytoday.com/blog/radical-teaching/201005/want-children-pay-attention-make-their-brains-curious

Winebrenner, S. (1992). *Teaching gifted kids in the regular classroom.* Minneapolis, MN: Free Spirit.

Wolfe, P. (2001). *Brain matters: Translating research into classroom practice.* Alexandria, VA: Association for Supervision and Curriculum Development.

Wolfe, P., & Sorgen, M. (1990). *Mind, memory and learning: Implications for the classroom.* Napa, CA: Author.

Wormeli, R. (2006). Fair isn't always equal: Assessing and grading in the differentiated classroom. Alexandria, VA: Association for Supervision and Curriculum Development.

Zull, J. (2002). *The art of changing the brain.* Sterling, VA: Stylus.

Index

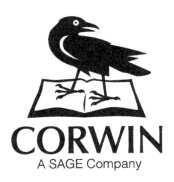

CORWIN

A SAGE Company

The Corwin logo—a raven striding across an open book—represents the union of courage and learning. Corwin is committed to improving education for all learners by publishing books and other professional development resources for those serving the field of PreK–12 education. By providing practical, hands-on materials, Corwin continues to carry out the promise of its motto: **"Helping Educators Do Their Work Better."**